Table of Contents

Table of Contents 1
Free Gift 7
Introduction 8
Breakfast Recipes 9
    Delicious Breakfast Pie 9
    Creamy Eggs and Turkey Mix 9
    Tasty Spinach Quiche 10
    Egg and Bacon Casserole 10
    Breakfast Omelet 11
    Healthy Veggie Casserole 11
    Mediterranean Frittata 12
    Delicious Egg Scramble 12
    Tasty Asparagus Casserole 13
    Tasty Asparagus and Mushroom Casserole 13
    Italian Eggs 14
    Incredible Turkey and Bacon Casserole 14
    Spinach and Feta Quiche 15
    Turkey Casserole 15
    Spicy Turkey and Eggs Mix 16
    Kale Frittata 16
    Beef Breakfast Bowl 17
    Salmon Omelet 17
    Mexican Pork Breakfast 18
    Beef and Bok Choy Mix 18
    Chorizo and Cauliflower Mix 19
    Salami and Eggs Casserole 19
    Simple Coconut Mix 20
    Beef and Radish Breakfast 20
    Eggs and Brussels Sprouts Breakfast 21
    Easy Chia Pudding 21
    Delicious Chicken Frittata 22
    Different Chicken Omelet 22
    Tomatoes Casserole 23
    Burrito Bowls 23
    Goat Cheese and Mushrooms Casserole 24
    Bell Pepper and Olives Frittata 24
    Squash and Zucchini Pudding 25
    Pear Breakfast Bowls 25
    Cauliflower Rice Pudding and Salsa 26
    Berry Butter 26
    Pumpkin Butter 27
    Cauliflower Rice Pudding 27
    Maple and Cauliflower Rice Pudding 28
    Fajita Bowls 28
    Pork Butt and Eggs Mix 29
    Leek, Kale and Turkey Breakfast 29

Meatloaf	30
Breakfast Veggies Mix	30
Butternut Squash Mix	31
Breakfast Pork and Avocado Mix	31
Breakfast Pork Salad	32
Sour Apples and Strawberries Breakfast Mix	32
Cauliflower and Mushroom Bowls	33
Turkey, Cranberries and Cauliflower Bowls	33
Main Dish Recipes	34
Delicious Pork Chili	34
Spiced Pork Ribs	34
Delicious Pork Stew	35
Simple Kalua Pork	35
Tasty Pork Shanks	36
Simple Bacon and Collard Greens	36
Simple Pork and Cauliflower Rice	37
Chili Verde	37
Tender Pork Loin	38
Corned Beef Brisket	38
Simple Beef Stew	39
Spicy Curry	39
Beef and Cabbage Stew	40
Beef and Veggie Stew	40
Red Curry	41
Tasty Meatballs	41
Simple Shredded Beef	42
American Beef Brisket	42
Mexican Beef Stew	43
Indian Beef Mix	43
Beef Tongue Mix	44
Ground Beef Soup	44
Chicken Drumsticks	45
Special Chicken Soup	45
Delicious Slow Cooked Chicken	46
Delicious Bacon Chicken	46
Chicken Curry	47
Yellow Chicken Curry	47
Delicious Shrimp	48
Garlic Shrimp	48
Shrimp and Squash Mix	49
Simple Oxtail Stew	49
Lamb Leg	50
Rabbit Stew	50
Beef Roast Soup	51
Easy Lamb Curry	51
Lamb Shoulder Mix	52
Delicious Creamy Chicken	52
Creamy Salmon Soup	53
Shrimp Stew	53

Tasty Seafood Stew	54
Seafood Chowder	54
Maple Salmon with Broccoli and Cauliflower	55
Italian Shrimp	55
Thai Pompano with Leeks	56
Spicy Tuna Loin	56
Braised Squid	57
Salmon with Cilantro Sauce	57
Steamed Salmon	58
Creamy Clams	58
Side Dishes	59
Mexican Veggie Mix	59
Fresh Veggie Side Dish	59
Spinach and Squash Mix	60
Cauliflower and Broccoli Fresh Mix	60
Special Cauliflower Rice Mix	61
Rustic Mashed Cauliflower	61
Squash and Parsnips Mix	62
Summer Greenie Mix	62
Fall Veggie Mix	63
Eggplant and Kale Mix	63
Brussels Sprouts and Onions	64
Cabbage and Apples Side Dish	64
Simple Mushrooms Caps Side Dish	65
Zucchini and Squash Side Dish	65
Cheesy Green Beans	66
Herbed Mushrooms Mix	66
Brussels Sprouts and Bacon	67
Creamy Spinach	67
Okra and Mint	68
Napa Cabbage Mix	68
Garlicky Swiss Chard	69
Mushroom and Arugula Mix	69
Red Chard Mix	70
Kale Side Dish	70
Hungarian Cabbage Side Dish	71
Mushrooms Winter Mix	71
Balsamic Swiss Chard with Pine Nuts and Raisins	72
Balsamic Spinach and Chard	72
Cherry Tomatoes Side Dish	73
Squash Mash	73
Red Chard and Capers	74
Balsamic Kale	74
Simple Broccoli Side Dish	75
Fast and Creamy Fennel Mix	75
Colored Bell Peppers Mix	76
Broccoli and Tomatoes Mix	76
Bok Choy and Bacon Mix	77
Creamy Celery Side Dish	77

Stewed Celery Mix ... 78
Lemony Collard Greens ... 78
Collard Greens, Bacon and Tomatoes ... 79
Mustard Greens and Garlic ... 79
Cheesy Collard Greens ... 80
Spring Green Mix ... 80
Easy Asparagus ... 81
Spanish Spinach Mix ... 81
Squash and Swiss Chard Mix ... 82
Simple Cherry Tomatoes and Onion Mix ... 82
Creamy Eggplant and Tomatoes ... 83
Creamy Radish Mix ... 83

Snack and Appetizer Recipes ... 84
Simple Cashew Spread ... 84
Beef Party Rolls ... 84
Eggplant and Tomato Salsa ... 85
Squash and Cauliflower Spread ... 85
Mixed Veggies Spread ... 86
Cashew Hummus ... 86
Spinach and Chestnuts Dip ... 87
Bell Peppers Appetizer ... 87
Artichoke and Coconut Spread ... 88
Mushroom and Bell Peppers Spread ... 88
Chicken Wings Appetizer ... 89
Cod Sticks ... 89
Pecans Snack ... 90
Party Meatballs ... 90
Shrimp, Mussels and Clams Appetizer ... 91
Curried Shrimp Appetizer ... 91
Stuffed Chicken Breast Appetizer ... 92
Pecans Snack ... 92
Spicy Cauliflower Dip ... 93
Spicy Nuts Mix ... 93
Veggie Party Mix ... 94
Walnuts and Pumpkin Seeds Snack ... 94
Coconut Crab Spread ... 95
Tomato and Sweet Onion Dip ... 95
Mussels and Veggies Appetizer ... 96
Cheese Dip ... 96
Different Cream Cheese Dip ... 97
Zucchini and Tomato Dip ... 97
Zucchini Hummus ... 98
Beef Jerky Snack ... 98
Stuffed Mushrooms ... 99
Cheesy Party Wings ... 99
Chicken Rolls ... 100
Zucchini and Cheese Rolls ... 100
Salmon Cakes ... 101
Salmon Salsa ... 101

- Tuna Cakes 102
- Creole Shrimp Appetizer 102
- Octopus Salad 103
- Cod Appetizer Salad 103
- Hot Salmon Bites 104
- Salmon Salad 104
- Chili Dip 105
- Radish Dip 105
- Strawberry Dip 106
- Balsamic Mushrooms Dip 106
- Clams and Mussels Appetizer Salad 107
- Easy Clams Delight 107
- Artichokes Appetizer 108
- Endives Appetizer Salad 108

Dessert Recipes 109
- Cocoa Pudding 109
- Raspberry Bars 109
- Mascarpone and Berries Cream 110
- Simple Lemon Cake 110
- Berry Pudding 111
- Stewed Raspberries 111
- Almond and Cocoa Cake 112
- Pumpkin and Cauliflower Pudding 112
- Berries Marmalade 113
- Zucchini Cake 113
- Squash Dessert 114
- Pear Pudding 114
- Coconut Bars 115
- Berries and Cream Dessert 115
- Almonds and Coconut Granola 116
- Cherry Marmalade 116
- Simple Cauliflower Pudding 117
- Pumpkin Cake 117
- Strawberries and Blueberries Marmalade 118
- Lemon Marmalade 118
- Sour Apples Jam 119
- Rhubarb and Berries Marmalade 119
- Sweet Plums 120
- Fruit Bowls 120
- Sweet Strawberry Cream 121
- Sour Apple Stew 121
- Berry Pie 122
- Simple Lemon Pudding 122
- Stuffed Apples 123
- Chocolate Cake 123
- Stewed Pears 124
- Maple Pecans 124
- Plum and Cinnamon Mousse 125
- Passion Fruit Dessert Cream 125

Cherry and Cocoa Mousse	126
Grapefruit and Mint Sauce	126
Maplè Figs Stew	127
Special Apple Cake	127
Vanilla Espresso Cream	128
Lemon and Blackberries Cream	128
Stewed Figs	129
Carrot Cake	129
Strawberry Marmalade	130
Raspberry Cream	130
Dried Fruits Pudding	131
Avocado Cake	131
Ricotta and Dates Cake	132
Rhubarb Mousse	132
Squash Pudding	133
Chestnut Cream	133
Conclusion	134
Recipe Index	135

Free Gift

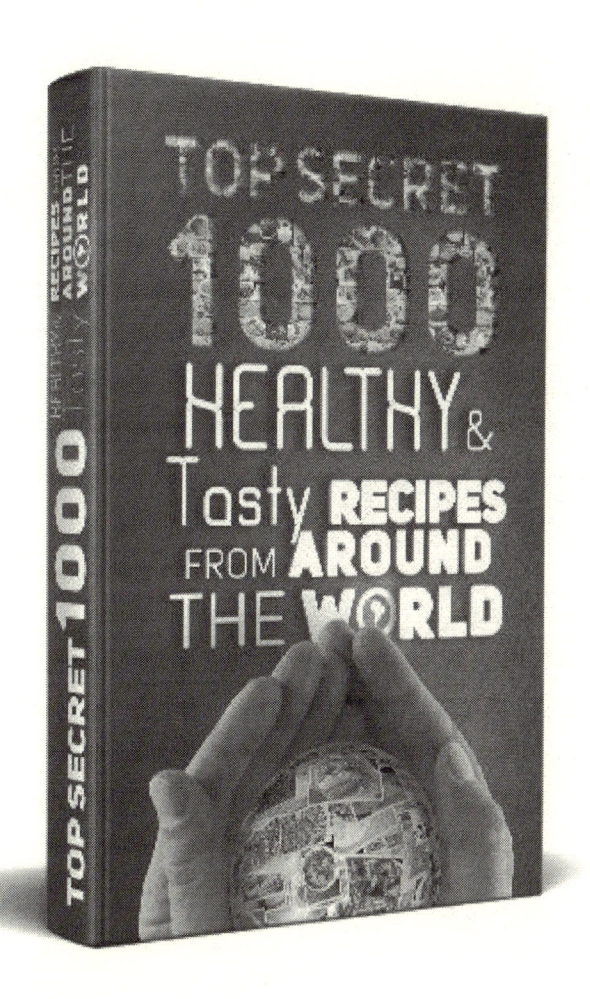

Up to 1000 delicious and healthy recipes from cooking traditions all around the world.

Please follow this link to get instant access to your Free Cookbook:
http://bookretailseller.pro/

Introduction

Are you looking for a healthy diet that brings you health benefits and improves your appearance at the same time? Do you want to make a change and to transform yourself into a new, healthier and happier person? Well, if the answer is "yes" to all these questions, you are definitely in the right place!

We searched for the best dietary option and we discover the Ketogenic diet!
This great diet is easy to follow and it will bring you all the benefits you are looking for!

The Ketogenic diet is a low carb one and the best thing about it is that it's very permissive.
If you choose such a diet, you need to know that you can eat a lot of veggies, greens, meat, eggs, nuts, seeds, healthy oils, cheese and berries.
On the other hand, if you opt for a keto diet, you have to stop consuming all kind of grains, sugar, beans, potatoes and other starchy foods.
So, as you can see for yourself, a Ketogenic diet is so easy to follow!

Now that you've made the decision to start a keto life, we recommend you to try something else as well.
We recommend you to cook all your new Ketogenic recipes in the best kitchen pot available on the market these days: In your slow cooker!
Trust us! Your keto meals with taste so great if you make them in your slow cooker!
All your meals with be so delicious, rich, textured and flavored!

So, what do you say?
Are you ready to start your new culinary adventure?
Have fun cooking your keto meals in your slow cooker!

Breakfast Recipes

Delicious Breakfast Pie

Preparation time: 10 minutes
Cooking time: 8 hours
Servings: 4

Ingredients:
- 8 eggs, whisked
- 1 yellow onion, chopped
- 1 pound boiled turkey fillet, chopped
- 2 teaspoons basil, dried
- 1 tablespoon garlic powder
- A pinch of salt and black pepper
- 1 yellow bell pepper, chopped
- A drizzle of olive oil

Directions:
Grease your Crockpot with the oil, add eggs, onion, turkey, basil, garlic powder, salt, pepper and yellow bell pepper, toss, cover and cook on Low for 8 hours. Slice, divide between plates and serve for breakfast. Enjoy!

Nutrition: calories 251, fat 4, fiber 4, carbs 6, protein 7

Creamy Eggs and Turkey Mix

Preparation time: 10 minutes
Cooking time: 5 hours
Servings: 4

Ingredients:
- 2 garlic cloves, minced
- A pinch of salt and black pepper
- 10 eggs, whisked
- 1 cup cheddar cheese, shredded
- ¾ cup whipping cream
- 12 ounces boiled turkey fillet, sliced
- 1 broccoli head, florets separated and roughly chopped
- A drizzle of olive oil

Directions:
Grease your Crockpot with the oil, add half of the broccoli, turkey and cheese. Add the rest of the broccoli, turkey and cheese. In a bowl, mix the eggs with whipping cream, salt, pepper and garlic, whisk and pour into the pot as well. Cover, cook on Low for 5 hours, divide between plates and serve for breakfast. Enjoy!

Nutrition: calories 211, fat 7, fiber 4, carbs 5, protein 5

Tasty Spinach Quiche

Preparation time: 10 minutes
Cooking time: 4 hours
Servings: 4

Ingredients:
- 10 ounces spinach
- 2 cups baby Bella mushrooms, chopped
- 1 red bell pepper, chopped
- 1 and ½ cups cheddar cheese, shredded
- 8 eggs
- 1 cup coconut cream
- 2 tablespoons chives, chopped
- A pinch of salt and black pepper
- ½ cup almond flour
- ¼ teaspoons baking soda
- Cooking spray

Directions:
In a bowl, mix the eggs with coconut cream, chives, salt and pepper and whisk. Add almond flour and baking soda and whisk well again. Add cheddar, bell pepper, mushrooms and spinach, toss, transfer to your Crockpot after you've greased it with cooking spray, cover and cook on Low for 4 hours. Slice quiche, divide between plates and serve for breakfast.
Enjoy!

Nutrition: calories 211, fat 6, fiber 6, carbs 6, protein 10

Egg and Bacon Casserole

Preparation time: 10 minutes
Cooking time: 4 hours
Servings: 6

Ingredients:
- 2 cups cheddar cheese, grated
- 1 and ½ cups bacon, cooked and crumbled
- 1 and ½ cups cherry tomatoes, halved
- 1 bunch scallions, chopped
- 1 tablespoon olive oil
- A pinch of salt and black pepper
- 8 eggs
- ½ cup coconut milk

Directions:
In a large bowl, mix the eggs with salt, pepper, milk, scallions, tomatoes, bacon and cheese and whisk well. Add the oil to your Crockpot, add eggs mix, cover and cook on Low for 4 hours. Divide between plates and serve.
Enjoy!

Nutrition: calories 172, fat 5, fiber 4, carbs 6, protein 8

Breakfast Omelet

Preparation time: 10 minutes
Cooking time: 3 hours
Servings: 4

Ingredients:
- Cooking spray
- 6 eggs
- 1 tablespoon coconut milk
- ½ red bell pepper, chopped
- ½ green bell pepper, chopped
- 1 small yellow onion, chopped
- ½ cup ham, chopped
- 1 cup cheddar cheese, shredded
- A pinch of salt and black pepper

Directions:
Grease your Crockpot with cooking spray and spread onion, ham, red and green bell pepper on the bottom. In a bowl, mix the eggs with salt, pepper, cheese and milk, whisk well and pour over veggies and ham. Cover, cook on High for 3 hours, divide between plates and serve for breakfast right away.
Enjoy!

Nutrition: calories 192, fat 6, fiber 5, carbs 6, protein 12

Healthy Veggie Casserole

Preparation time: 10 minutes
Cooking time: 4 hours
Servings: 8

Ingredients:
- 8 eggs
- 4 egg whites
- 2 teaspoons mustard
- ¾ cup almond milk
- A pinch of salt and black pepper
- 2 red bell peppers, chopped
- 1 yellow onion, chopped
- 1 teaspoon sweet paprika
- 4 bacon strips, chopped
- 6 ounces cheddar cheese, shredded
- Cooking spray

Directions:
In a bowl, mix the eggs with egg whites, mustard, milk, salt, pepper and sweet paprika and whisk well. Grease your Crockpot with cooking spray and spread bell peppers, bacon and onion on the bottom. Add mixed eggs, sprinkle cheddar all over, cover and cook on Low for 4 hours. Divide between plates and serve for breakfast.
Enjoy!

Nutrition: calories 172, fat 6, fiber 3, carbs 6, protein 7

Mediterranean Frittata

Preparation time: 10 minutes
Cooking time: 4 hours
Servings: 4

Ingredients:
- 8 eggs
- A pinch of salt and black pepper
- ½ cup coconut milk
- 1 teaspoon oregano, dried
- 4 cups baby arugula
- 1 and ¼ cup roasted red peppers, chopped
- ½ cup red onion, chopped
- ¾ cup goat cheese, crumbled
- Cooking spray

Directions:
In a bowl, mix the eggs with milk, oregano, salt and pepper and whisk well. Grease your Crockpot with cooking spray and spread roasted peppers, onion and arugula on the bottom. Add eggs mix, sprinkle goat cheese all over, cover and cook on Low for 4 hours. Divide frittata between plates and serve for breakfast. Enjoy!

Nutrition: calories 199, fat 3, fiber 6, carbs 6, protein 4

Delicious Egg Scramble

Preparation time: 10 minutes
Cooking time: 6 hours
Servings: 6

Ingredients:
- 12 eggs
- 14 ounces boiled turkey fillet, sliced
- 1 cup coconut milk
- 16 ounces cheddar cheese, shredded
- A pinch of salt and black pepper
- 1 teaspoon basil, dried
- 1 teaspoon oregano, dried
- Cooking spray

Directions:
Grease your Crockpot with cooking spray and spread turkey meat on the bottom. Crack eggs, add milk, basil, oregano, salt and pepper, whisk a bit, sprinkle cheddar all over, cover and cook on Low for 6 hours. Divide egg scramble between plates and serve.
Enjoy!

Nutrition: calories 177, fat 4, fiber 5, carbs 6, protein 9

Tasty Asparagus Casserole

Preparation time: 10 minutes
Cooking time: 6 hours
Servings: 4

Ingredients:
- 10 ounces cream of celery
- 12 ounces asparagus, chopped
- 2 eggs, hard- boiled, peeled and sliced
- 1 cup cheddar cheese, shredded
- 1 teaspoon olive oil

Directions:
Grease your Crockpot with the oil. Add cream of celery and cheese to the pot and stir. Add asparagus and eggs, cover and cook on Low for 6 hours. Divide between plates and serve for breakfast.
Enjoy!

Nutrition: calories 241, fat 5, fiber 4, carbs 5, protein 12

Tasty Asparagus and Mushroom Casserole

Preparation time: 10 minutes
Cooking time: 5 hours
Servings: 4

Ingredients:
- 2 pounds asparagus spears, cut into medium pieces
- 1 cup mushrooms, sliced
- A drizzle of olive oil
- A pinch of salt and black pepper
- 2 cups coconut milk
- 1 teaspoon soy sauce
- 5 eggs, whisked

Directions:
Grease your Crockpot with the oil and spread asparagus and mushrooms on the bottom. In a bowl, mix the eggs with milk, salt, pepper and soy sauce, whisk, pour into the pot, toss everything, cover and cook on Low for 6 hours. Divide between plates and serve right away for breakfast.
Enjoy!

Nutrition: calories 211, fat 4, fiber 4, carbs 6, protein 5

Italian Eggs

Preparation time: 10 minutes
Cooking time: 6 hours
Servings: 4

Ingredients:
- 1 and ½ tablespoon olive oil
- 1 yellow onion, chopped
- 3 garlic cloves, minced
- 27 ounces canned tomatoes, crushed
- 1 tablespoon soy sauce
- 2 tablespoons fresh tomato puree
- 1 teaspoon basil, dried
- 1 teaspoon oregano, dried
- ¼ teaspoon chili flakes
- A pinch of salt and black pepper
- 4 eggs
- ¼ cup parsley, chopped

Directions:
Heat up a pan with the oil over medium heat, add garlic and onion, stir, cook for 2-3 minutes and transfer everything to your Crockpot. Add tomatoes, fresh tomato puree, soy sauce, chili flakes, oregano, basil, salt and pepper, cover and cook on Low for 6 hours. Make 4 well In this mix, crack an egg In each, cover and cook on High for 20 minutes more. Sprinkle parsley all over, divide everything between plates and serve for breakfast.
Enjoy!

Nutrition: calories 222, fat 4, fiber 6, carbs 6, protein 10

Incredible Turkey and Bacon Casserole

Preparation time: 10 minutes
Cooking time: 3 hours
Servings: 4

Ingredients:
- 6 bacon slices, chopped
- 10 oz turkey, sliced
- 6 oz butternut squash, chopped
- 2 tablespoons fresh tomato puree
- 1 teaspoon sweet paprika
- 2 leeks, chopped
- 10 ounces canned tomatoes, chopped
- 3 ounces water
- A pinch of salt and black pepper

Directions:
In your Crockpot, mix bacon with turkey, squash, fresh tomato puree, paprika, leeks, tomatoes, water, salt and pepper, toss, cover and cook on High for 3 hours. Divide between plates and serve for breakfast.
Enjoy!

Nutrition: calories 217, fat 6, fiber 5, carbs 6, protein 16

Spinach and Feta Quiche

Preparation time: 10 minutes
Cooking time: 6 hours
Servings: 8

Ingredients:
- 1 pound chicken, ground
- 10 ounces spinach
- 6 ounces feta cheese, crumbled
- 1/3 cup dill, chopped
- 2 tablespoons onion flakes
- 6 eggs
- 12 ounces coconut milk
- A pinch of salt and black pepper
- Cooking spray

Directions:
Grease your Crockpot with cooking spray. In a bowl, mix chicken with feta, spinach, dill, onion flakes, salt and pepper and stir well. In a separate bowl, mix the eggs with salt, pepper and milk and whisk well. Add this to chicken mix, toss everything, transfer to your Crockpot, cover and cook on Low for 6 hours. Divide between plates and serve for breakfast.
Enjoy!

Nutrition: calories 251, fat 5, fiber 5, carbs 6, protein 18

Turkey Casserole

Preparation time: 10 minutes
Cooking time: 4 hours
Servings: 8

Ingredients:
- 1 pound turkey fillet, boiled, chopped
- 1 yellow onion, chopped
- 1 sweet red pepper, chopped
- 2 jalapenos, chopped
- 12 eggs
- 1 cup coconut milk
- ½ cup Mexican cheese, shredded
- A pinch of salt and white pepper
- Cooking spray

Directions:
Heat up a pan over medium- high heat, add turkey, jalapenos, red pepper and onion, stir, cook for 7 minutes and transfer to your Crockpot after you've greased it with cooking spray. In a bowl, mix the eggs with salt, pepper and milk, whisk well and pour over turkey mix. Sprinkle cheese, cover pot and cook on Low for 4 hours. Divide between plates and serve hot.
Enjoy!

Nutrition: calories 272, fat 6, fiber 4, carbs 7, protein 22

Spicy Turkey and Eggs Mix

Preparation time: 10 minutes
Cooking time: 5 hours
Servings: 3

Ingredients:
- A drizzle of olive oil
- ¼ pound boiled turkey fillet, chopped
- ¼ cup green onions, chopped
- A pinch of salt and black pepper
- 6 eggs
- 1 tablespoon cilantro, chopped

Directions:
Heat up a pan with the oil over medium- high heat, add turkey meat, stir, cook for 6-7 minutes and transfer to your Crockpot. In a bowl, mix the eggs with salt, pepper, green onions and cilantro, whisk well, pour over turkey meat, cover pot and cook on Low for 5 hours. Divide between plates and serve for breakfast.
Enjoy!

Nutrition: calories 261, fat 6, fiber 6, carbs 8, protein 22

Kale Frittata

Preparation time: 10 minutes
Cooking time: 3 hours
Servings: 4

Ingredients:
- 1 teaspoon olive oil
- 7 ounces roasted red peppers, chopped
- 6 ounces baby kale
- 6 ounces feta cheese, crumbled
- ¼ cup green onions, sliced
- 7 eggs, whisked
- A pinch of salt and black pepper

Directions:
In a bowl, mix the eggs with cheese, kale, red peppers, green onions, salt and pepper, whisk well and pour into the Crockpot after you've greased it with the oil. Cover pot, cook on Low for 3 hours, divide between plates and serve right away.
Enjoy!

Nutrition: calories 261, fat 7, fiber 4, carbs 6, protein 16

Beef Breakfast Bowl

Preparation time: 10 minutes
Cooking time: 4 hours
Servings: 2

Ingredients:

- 4 ounces beef, ground
- 1 yellow onion, chopped
- 8 mushrooms, sliced
- A pinch of salt and black pepper
- 2 eggs, whisked
- 1 tablespoon olive oil
- ½ teaspoon smoked paprika
- 1 avocado, pitted, peeled and chopped
- 12 black olives, pitted and sliced

Directions:
Drizzle the oil In your Crockpot, add onions, mushrooms, beef, salt, pepper and smoked paprika and stir. Add whisked eggs, stir, cover and cook on Low for 4 hours. Divide beef mix into bowls, top each with avocado and black olives and serve for breakfast.
Enjoy!

Nutrition: calories 260, fat 13, fiber 4, carbs 6, protein 43

Salmon Omelet

Preparation time: 10 minutes
Cooking time: 3 hours and 40 minutes
Servings: 3

Ingredients:

- 4 eggs, whisked
- ½ teaspoon olive oil
- A pinch of salt and black pepper
- 4 ounces smoked salmon, chopped

For the sauce:

- 1 cup almond milk
- ½ cup cashews, soaked, drained
- ¼ cup green onions, chopped
- 1 teaspoon garlic powder
- Salt and black pepper to the taste
- 1 tablespoon lemon juice

Directions:
In your blender, mix cashews with milk, garlic powder, lemon juice, green onions, salt and pepper, blend really well and leave aside for now. Drizzle the oil In your Crockpot, add eggs, salt and pepper, whisk, cover and cook on Low for 3 hours. Add salmon, toss a bit, cover, cook on Low for 40 minutes more and divide between plates. Drizzle green onions sauce all over and serve for breakfast.
Enjoy!

Nutrition: calories 200, fat 10, fiber 2, carbs 6, protein 15

Mexican Pork Breakfast

Preparation time: 10 minutes
Cooking time: 5 hours
Servings: 8

Ingredients:
- 3 oz Mexican chilis
- 1 pound pork, ground
- 1 pound turkey, boiled, chopped
- Salt and black pepper to the taste
- 8 eggs, whisked eggs
- 1 tomato, chopped
- 3 tablespoons olive oil
- ½ cup red onion, chopped
- 1 avocado, pitted, peeled and chopped

Directions:
In a bowl, mix pork with turkey, stir and spread on the bottom of your Crockpot after you've greased it with the oil. Add Mexican chilis, cover and cook on Low for 3 hours. Add eggs, tomato, onion, salt and pepper, toss well, cover and cook on High for 2 hours more. Divide pork and eggs on plates, add avocado on top and serve.
Enjoy!

Nutrition: calories 400, fat 15, fiber 4, carbs 7, protein 25

Beef and Bok Choy Mix

Preparation time: 10 minutes
Cooking time: 5 hours
Servings: 2

Ingredients:
- ½ pounds beef meat, minced
- 2 teaspoons red chili flakes
- 1 tablespoon tamari sauce
- 2 bell peppers, chopped
- 1 teaspoon chili powder
- 2 tablespoons olive oil
- A pinch of salt and black pepper
- 6 bunches bok choy, trimmed and chopped
- 1 teaspoon ginger, grated

Directions:
Heat up a pan with 1 tablespoon oil over medium- high heat, add beef and bell peppers, stir, cook for 10 minutes and transfer to your Crockpot. Add chili flakes, tamari sauce, chili powder, salt, pepper, bok choy, ginger and the rest of the oil, stir, cover and cook on Low for 5 hours. Divide between bowls and serve for breakfast.
Enjoy!

Nutrition: calories 248, fat 14, fiber 4, carbs 7, protein 14

Chorizo and Cauliflower Mix

Preparation time: 10 minutes
Cooking time: 5 hours
Servings: 4

Ingredients:
- 1 pound chorizo, chopped
- 12 ounces canned green chilies, chopped
- 1 yellow onion, chopped
- ½ teaspoon garlic powder
- A pinch of salt and black pepper
- 1 cauliflower head, florets separated and riced
- 4 eggs, whisked
- 2 tablespoons green onions, chopped

Directions:
Heat up a pan over medium heat, add chorizo and onion, stir, brown for a few minutes and transfer to your Crockpot. Add chilies, garlic powder, salt, pepper, cauliflower, eggs and green onions, toss, cover and cook on Low for 5 hours. Divide between bowls and serve for breakfast.
Enjoy!

Nutrition: calories 350, fat 12, fiber 4, carbs 6, protein 20

Salami and Eggs Casserole

Preparation time: 10 minutes
Cooking time: 5 hours
Servings: 4

Ingredients:
- 2 tablespoons ghee, melted
- 2 zucchinis, sliced
- Salt and black pepper to the taste
- ½ cup tomatoes, chopped
- 2 garlic cloves, minced
- 1/3 cup yellow onion, chopped
- ½ teaspoon Italian seasoning
- 3 ounces Italian salami, chopped
- ½ cup kalamata olives, chopped
- 6 eggs, whisked
- 2 tablespoons parsley, chopped

Directions:
Heat up a pan with the ghee over medium heat, add garlic, onions, salt and pepper, stir, cook for a couple of minutes and transfer to your Crockpot. Add salami, tomatoes, zucchini, olives, Italian seasoning and eggs, toss everything a bit, cover and cook on Low for 5 hours. Add parsley, divide between plates and serve.
Enjoy!

Nutrition: calories 333, fat 23, fiber 4, carbs 12, protein 15

Simple Coconut Mix

Preparation time: 5 minutes
Cooking time: 3 hours
Servings: 1

Ingredients:
- 1 teaspoon cinnamon powder
- ½ teaspoon nutmeg, ground
- ½ cup almonds, ground
- 1 teaspoon stevia
- 1 and ½ cup coconut cream
- ¼ teaspoon cardamom, ground
- ¼ teaspoon cloves, ground

Directions:
In your Crockpot, mix coconut cream with cinnamon, nutmeg, almonds, stevia, cardamom and cloves, stir, cover and cook on Low for 3 hours. Divide between bowls and serve.
Enjoy!

Nutrition: calories 200, fat 12, fiber 4, carbs 8, protein 16

Beef and Radish Breakfast

Preparation time: 10 minutes
Cooking time: 3 hours
Servings: 2

Ingredients:
- 1 tablespoon olive oil
- 2 garlic cloves, minced
- ½ cup beef stock
- A pinch of salt and black pepper
- 1 yellow onion, chopped
- 2 cups corned beef, chopped
- 7 oz radishes, cut into quarters

Directions:
Drizzle the oil on the bottom of your Crockpot and add beef. Also add radishes, garlic, stock, onion, salt and pepper, toss, cover and cook on Low for 3 hours. Divide between bowls and serve right away for breakfast.
Enjoy!

Nutrition: calories 240, fat 7, fiber 3, carbs 7, protein 8

Eggs and Brussels Sprouts Breakfast

Preparation time: 10 minutes
Cooking time: 4 hours
Servings: 4

Ingredients:
- 4 eggs, whisked
- Salt and black pepper to the taste
- 1 tablespoon avocado oil
- 2 shallots, minced
- 2 garlic cloves, minced
- 12 ounces Brussels sprouts, sliced
- 2 ounces bacon, chopped

Directions:
Drizzle the oil on the bottom of your Crockpot and spread Brussels sprouts, garlic, bacon and shallots on the bottom. Add whisked eggs, salt and pepper, toss, cover and cook on Low for 4 hours. Divide between plates and serve right away for breakfast.
Enjoy!

Nutrition: calories 240, fat 7, fiber 4, carbs 7, protein 13

Easy Chia Pudding

Preparation time: 10 minutes
Cooking time: 3 hours and 15 minutes
Servings: 2

Ingredients:
- 2 tablespoons coffee
- 2 cups water
- 1/3 cup chia seeds
- 1 tablespoon stevia
- 1 tablespoon vanilla extract
- 2 tablespoons unsweetened chocolate chips
- ¼ cup coconut cream

Directions:
Heat up a small pot with the water over medium heat, bring to a boil, add coffee, simmer for 15 minutes, take off heat and strain Into your Crockpot. Add vanilla extract, coconut cream, stevia, chocolate chips and chia seeds, stir well, cover and cook on Low for 3 hours. Divide between bowls and serve cold for breakfast.
Enjoy!

Nutrition: calories 100, fat 0.4, fiber 4, carbs 3, protein 3

Delicious Chicken Frittata

Preparation time: 10 minutes
Cooking time: 5 hours
Servings: 5

Ingredients:
- 7 eggs
- 3 tablespoons almond flour
- 1 tablespoon olive oil
- A pinch of salt and black pepper
- 2 zucchinis, grated
- ½ cup coconut cream
- 1 teaspoon fennel seeds
- 1 teaspoon oregano, dried
- 1 pound chicken meat, ground

Directions:
In a bowl, mix the eggs with flour, salt, pepper, cream, zucchini, fennel, oregano and meat, whisk well, pour Into your Crockpot after you've greased it with the oil, cover and cook on Low for 5 hours. Slice frittata, divide between plates and serve for breakfast.
Enjoy!

Nutrition: calories 300, fat 23, fiber 3, carbs 4, protein 18

Different Chicken Omelet

Preparation time: 10 minutes
Cooking time: 3 hours
Servings: 2

Ingredients:
- 1 ounce rotisserie chicken, shredded
- 1 teaspoon mustard
- 1 tablespoon homemade mayonnaise
- 1 tomato, chopped
- 2 bacon slices, cooked and crumbled
- 4 eggs
- 1 small avocado, pitted, peeled and chopped
- Salt and black pepper to the taste

Directions:
In a bowl, mix the eggs with salt and pepper and whisk. Add chicken, avocado, tomato, bacon, mayo and mustard, toss, transfer to your Crockpot, cover and cook on Low for 3 hours. Divide between plates and serve.
Enjoy!

Nutrition: calories 270, fat 32, fiber 6, carbs 4, protein 25

Tomatoes Casserole

Preparation time: 10 minutes
Cooking time: 4 hours
Servings: 4

Ingredients:
- 2 teaspoons onion powder
- ¾ cup cashews, soaked for 30 minutes and drained
- 1 teaspoon garlic powder
- ½ teaspoon sage, dried
- Salt and black pepper to the taste
- 1 yellow onion, chopped
- 2 tablespoons parsley, chopped
- 3 garlic cloves, minced
- 1 tablespoon olive oil
- 5 tomatoes, cubed
- ½ teaspoon red pepper flakes

Directions:
In your blender, mix cashews with onion powder, garlic powder, sage, salt and pepper and pulse really well. Add oil to your Crockpot and arrange tomatoes, pepper flakes, garlic, onion, salt, pepper and parsley. Add cashews sauce, toss, cover, cook on High for 4 hours, divide between plates and serve for breakfast.
Enjoy!

Nutrition: calories 218, fat 6, fiber 6, carbs 6, protein 5

Burrito Bowls

Preparation time: 10 minutes
Cooking time: 6 hours
Servings: 6

Ingredients:
- 10 ounces feta cheese, crumbled
- 1 green bell pepper, chopped
- ¼ cup scallions, chopped
- 15 ounces canned tomatoes, chopped
- 1 cup fresh tomato puree
- ½ cup water
- ¼ teaspoon cumin powder
- ½ teaspoon turmeric powder
- ½ teaspoon smoked paprika
- A pinch of salt and black pepper
- ¼ teaspoon chili powder
- 3 cups spinach leaves, torn

Directions:
In your Crockpot, mix cheese with bell pepper, scallions, tomatoes, tomato puree, water, cumin, turmeric, paprika, salt, pepper and chili powder, stir, cover and cook on Low for 6 hours. Add spinach, toss well, divide this Into bowls and serve for breakfast.
Enjoy!

Nutrition: calories 211, fat 4, fiber 7, carbs 7, protein 4

Goat Cheese and Mushrooms Casserole

Preparation time: 10 minutes
Cooking time: 4 hours
Servings: 4

Ingredients:
- 1 teaspoon lemon zest, grated
- 10 ounces goat cheese, cubed
- 1 tablespoon lemon juice
- 1 tablespoon apple cider vinegar
- 1 tablespoon olive oil
- 2 garlic cloves, minced
- 10 ounces spinach, torn
- ½ cup yellow onion, chopped
- ½ teaspoon basil, dried
- 8 ounces mushrooms, sliced
- A pinch of salt and black pepper
- ¼ teaspoon red pepper flakes
- Cooking spray

Directions:
Spray your Crockpot with cooking spray and arrange cheese cubes on the bottom. Add lemon zest, lemon juice, vinegar, olive oil, garlic, spinach, onion, basil, mushrooms, salt, pepper and pepper flakes, toss well, cover and cook on Low for 4 hours. Divide between plates and serve for breakfast right away.
Enjoy!

Nutrition: calories 216, fat 6, fiber 5, carbs 7, protein 4

Bell Pepper and Olives Frittata

Preparation time: 10 minutes
Cooking time: 6 hours
Servings: 4

Ingredients:
- 1 pound goat cheese, crumbled
- 2 tablespoons olive oil
- 1 yellow onion, chopped
- ¼ teaspoon turmeric powder
- 3 tablespoons garlic, minced
- 4 eggs, whisked
- 3 red bell peppers, chopped
- A pinch of salt and black pepper
- ½ cup kalamata olives, pitted and halved
- 1 teaspoon basil, dried
- 1 teaspoon oregano, dried
- 1 tablespoon lemon juice

Directions:
Add the oil to your Crockpot, spread cheese all over, add onion, turmeric, garlic, bell pepper, olives, basil, oregano, lemon juice, eggs, salt and pepper, toss a bit, cover and cook on Low for 6 hours. Divide between plates and serve for breakfast.
Enjoy!

Nutrition: calories 271, fat 4, fiber 5, carbs 7, protein 6

Squash and Zucchini Pudding

Preparation time: 10 minutes
Cooking time: 8 hours
Servings: 4

Ingredients:
- 5 oz butternut squash, grated
- 1 and ½ cups almond milk
- 1 zucchini, grated
- A pinch of nutmeg, ground
- A pinch of cloves, ground
- ½ teaspoon cinnamon powder
- 2 tablespoons sugar-free maple syrup
- ¼ cup walnuts, chopped
- 1 teaspoon vanilla extract

Directions:
In your Crockpot, mix squash with zucchini, milk, cloves, nutmeg, cinnamon, sugar-free maple syrup, walnuts and vanilla extract, stir, cover and cook on Low for 8 hours. Divide between bowls and serve for breakfast.
Enjoy!

Nutrition: calories 215, fat 4, fiber 4, carbs 7, protein 7

Pear Breakfast Bowls

Preparation time: 10 minutes
Cooking time: 9 hours
Servings: 2

Ingredients:
- 1 pear, cored and chopped
- ½ teaspoon maple extract
- 2 cups coconut milk
- ½ cup flax meal
- ½ teaspoon vanilla extract
- 1 tablespoon stevia
- ¼ cup walnuts, chopped
- Cooking spray

Directions:
Spray your Crockpot with some cooking spray, add coconut milk, maple extract, flax meal, pear, stevia and vanilla extract, stir, cover and cook on Low for 9 hours. Divide it Into breakfast bowls and serve with chopped walnuts on top.
Enjoy!

Nutrition: calories 150, fat 3, fiber 2, carbs 6, protein 6

Cauliflower Rice Pudding and Salsa

Preparation time: 10 minutes
Cooking time: 2 hours
Servings: 4

Ingredients:
- 1 cup cauliflower, riced
- ½ cup onion, chopped
- 1 cup veggie stock
- 1 red bell pepper, chopped
- 1 green bell pepper, chopped
- 4 ounces canned green chilies, chopped
- A pinch of salt and black pepper
- 1 avocado, pitted, peeled and cubed
- ½ cup cilantro, chopped
- ½ cup green onions, chopped
- ½ cup tomato, chopped
- 1 poblano pepper, chopped
- 2 tablespoons olive oil
- ½ teaspoon cumin, ground

For the salsa:
- 3 tablespoons lime juice

Directions:
In your Crockpot, mix cauliflower with stock and onions, stir, cover and cook on High for 1 hour and 30 minutes. Add chilies, red and green bell peppers, salt and pepper, stir, cover again and cook on High for 30 minutes more. Meanwhile, In a bowl, mix avocado with green onions, tomato, poblano pepper, cilantro, oil, cumin, a pinch of salt, black pepper and lime juice and stir really well. Divide rice mix Into bowls, top each with the salsa and serve.
Enjoy!

Nutrition: calories 140, fat 2, fiber 2, carbs 5, protein 5

Berry Butter

Preparation time: 10 minutes
Cooking time: 5 hours
Servings: 10

Ingredients:
- 5 cups blueberry puree
- 2 teaspoons cinnamon powder
- Zest of 1 lemon, grated
- 1/3 cup erythritol
- ½ teaspoon nutmeg powder
- ¼ teaspoon ginger powder

Directions:
Put blueberries in your slow cooker, cover and cook on Low for 4 hours. Add erythritol, ginger, nutmeg and lemon zest, stir and cook on High uncovered for 1 hour more. Divide Into jars and serve for breakfast whenever.
Enjoy!

Nutrition: calories 143, fat 2, fiber 3, carbs 3, protein 4

Pumpkin Butter

Preparation time: 10 minutes
Cooking time: 4 hours
Servings: 5

Ingredients:
- 2 teaspoons cinnamon powder
- 4 cups pumpkin puree
- 1 and ¼ cup sugar-free maple syrup
- ½ teaspoon nutmeg
- 1 teaspoon vanilla extract

Directions:
In your Crockpot, mix pumpkin puree with sugar-free maple syrup, vanilla extract, cinnamon and nutmeg, stir, cover and cook on High for 4 hours. Divide Into jars and serve for breakfast!
Enjoy!

Nutrition: calories 120, fat 2, fiber 2, carbs 4, protein 2

Cauliflower Rice Pudding

Preparation time: 10 minutes
Cooking time: 3 hours
Servings: 2

Ingredients:
- 4 tablespoons stevia
- 2 cups almond milk
- 1 cup cauliflower rice
- 1 teaspoon vanilla extract
- 1 tablespoons flaxseed meal
- 1 teaspoon cinnamon powder

Directions:
In your Crockpot, mix almond milk with stevia, cauliflower rice, vanilla, flaxseed meal, and cinnamon, stir, cover and cook on Low for 2 hours. Stir your pudding again, cover, cook on Low for 1 more hour, divide between bowls and serve for breakfast.
Enjoy!

Nutrition: calories 160, fat 2, fiber 3, carbs 8, protein 12

Maple and Cauliflower Rice Pudding

Preparation time: 10 minutes
Cooking time: 2 hours
Servings: 2

Ingredients:
- ¼ cup sugar-free maple syrup
- 3 cups almond milk
- 1 cup cauliflower rice
- 2 tablespoons vanilla extract

Directions:
Put cauliflower rice In your Crockpot, add sugar-free maple syrup, almond milk and vanilla extract, stir, cover and cook on High for 2 hours. Stir your pudding again, divide between bowls and serve for breakfast. Enjoy!

Nutrition: calories 140, fat 2, fiber 2, carbs 5, protein 5

Fajita Bowls

Preparation time: 10 minutes
Cooking time: 2 hours
Servings: 8

Ingredients:
- 4 ounces canned green chilies, chopped
- 3 tomatoes, chopped
- 1 green bell pepper, chopped
- 1 yellow onion, chopped
- 1 red bell pepper, chopped
- 2 teaspoons cumin, ground
- ½ teaspoon oregano, dried
- 2 teaspoons chili powder
- A pinch of salt and black pepper
- 2 avocados, pitted, peeled and chopped
- Cooking spray

Directions:
Grease your Crockpot with cooking spray, add chilies, tomatoes, bell peppers, onion, cumin, oregano, chili powder, salt and pepper, stir, cover and cook on High for 2 hours. Stir again, divide veggies mix Into bowls add avocado on top and serve for breakfast
Enjoy!

Nutrition: calories 140, fat 3, fiber 2, carbs 8, protein 12

Pork Butt and Eggs Mix

Preparation time: 10 minutes
Cooking time: 8 hours
Servings: 4

Ingredients:
- 1 medium pork butt
- 1 teaspoon coriander, ground
- 1 tablespoon oregano, dried
- 1 tablespoon cumin powder
- 2 tablespoons chili powder
- 1 onion, chopped
- A pinch of salt and black pepper
- 1 teaspoon lime juice
- 4 eggs, already fried
- 2 avocados, peeled, pitted and sliced

Directions:
In a bowl, mix pork butt with coriander, oregano, cumin, chili powder, onions and a pinch of black pepper, rub well, transfer to your slow cooker and cook on Low for 8 hours. Shred meat, divide between plates and serve for breakfast with fried eggs and avocado slices on top and with lime juice drizzled at the end
Enjoy!

Nutrition: calories 220, fat 2, fiber 2, carbs 6, protein 2

Leek, Kale and Turkey Breakfast

Preparation time: 10 minutes
Cooking time: 6 hours
Servings: 4

Ingredients:
- 1 and 1/3 cups leek, chopped
- 2 tablespoons olive oil
- 1 cup kale, chopped
- 2 teaspoons garlic, minced
- 8 eggs, whisked
- 1 and ½ cups boiled turkey fillet, chopped

Directions:
Heat up a pan with the oil over medium- high heat, add leek, garlic and kale, stir, cook for 2 minutes and transfer to your Crockpot. Add eggs and turkey meat, stir everything, cover and cook on Low for 6 hours. Slice, divide between plates and serve for breakfast.
Enjoy!

Nutrition: calories 220, fat 2, fiber 2, carbs 6, protein 10

Meatloaf

Preparation time: 10 minutes
Cooking time: 3 hours
Servings: 4

Ingredients:

- 1 onion, chopped
- 2 pounds pork, minced
- 1 teaspoon red pepper flakes, crushed
- 1 teaspoon olive oil
- 3 garlic cloves, minced
- ¼ cup almond flour
- 1 teaspoon oregano, chopped
- 1 tablespoon sage, minced
- A pinch of salt and black pepper
- 1 tablespoon sweet paprika
- 1 teaspoon marjoram, dried
- 2 eggs

Directions:
Heat up a pan with the oil over medium-high heat, add onion and garlic, stir, cook for 2 minutes and leave aside to cool down. In a bowl, mix pork with salt, pepper, pepper flakes, flour, oregano, sage, paprika, marjoram, eggs, garlic and onion and whisk everything. Shape your meatloaf, transfer to your Crockpot, cover and cook on Low for 3 hours. Leave aside to cool down, slice and serve for breakfast.
Enjoy!

Nutrition: calories 200, fat 3, fiber 2, carbs 7, protein 10

Breakfast Veggies Mix

Preparation time: 10 minutes
Cooking time: 3 hours
Servings: 4

Ingredients:

- ½ cup red onion, cut into medium chunks
- 1 cup cherry tomatoes, halved
- 2 and ½ cups zucchini, sliced
- 2 cups yellow bell pepper, chopped
- 1 cup mushrooms, sliced
- 2 tablespoons basil, chopped
- 1 tablespoon thyme, chopped
- ½ cup olive oil
- ½ cup balsamic vinegar

Directions:
In your Crockpot, mix onion pieces with tomatoes, zucchini, bell pepper, mushrooms, basil, thyme, oil and vinegar, toss to coat everything, cover and cook on High for 3 hours. Divide between plates and serve for breakfast.
Enjoy!

Nutrition: calories 150, fat 2, fiber 2, carbs 6, protein 5

Butternut Squash Mix

Preparation time: 10 minutes
Cooking time: 8 hours
Servings: 4

Ingredients:
- ½ cup walnuts, soaked for 12hours and drained
- ½ cup almonds
- 1 butternut squash, peeled and cubed
- 1 teaspoon cinnamon powder
- ½ teaspoon nutmeg, ground
- 1/3 tablespoon stevia
- 1 cup coconut milk

Directions:
In your Crockpot, mix walnuts with almonds, squash, cinnamon, nutmeg, stevia and milk, stir, cover and cook on Low for 8 hours. Divide between bowls and serve for breakfast.
Enjoy!

Nutrition: calories 202, fat 3, fiber 7, carbs 14, protein 2

Breakfast Pork and Avocado Mix

Preparation time: 10 minutes
Cooking time: 10 hours
Servings: 4

Ingredients:
- 4 pounds pork butt roast
- 1 tablespoon cumin powder
- 2 tablespoons chili powder
- 1 teaspoon coriander, ground
- 1 tablespoon oregano, dried
- 2 yellow onions, sliced
- 2 avocados, peeled, pitted and sliced

Directions:
In your slow cooker, mix pork butt with chili, cumin, oregano, coriander and onions, toss, cover and cook on Low for 10 hours. Shred meat, divide between plates, top with avocado slices and serve for breakfast.
Enjoy!

Nutrition: calories 270, fat 4, fiber 10, carbs 8, protein 25

Breakfast Pork Salad

Preparation time: 10 minutes
Cooking time: 10 hours
Servings: 4

Ingredients:
- 1 yellow onion, chopped
- 3 pounds pork shoulder
- 1 tablespoon cumin, ground
- 2 tablespoon smoked paprika
- 1 tablespoon chili powder
- 1 tablespoon garlic powder
- 2 teaspoons oregano, dried
- 1 teaspoon allspice, ground
- 1 teaspoon cinnamon powder
- A pinch of salt and black pepper
- Juice of 1 lemon
- 1 romaine lettuce head, leaves torn

Directions:
In your Crockpot, mix pork with onion, cumin, paprika, chili, garlic powder, oregano, allspice, cinnamon, salt, pepper and lemon juice, toss, cover and cook on Low for 10 hours. Shred meat using 2 forks, transfer to a bowl, add lettuce and some of the cooking liquid from the pot, toss, divide between plates and serve on a Sunday for breakfast.
Enjoy!

Nutrition: calories 261, fat 4, fiber 6, carbs 7, protein 29

Sour Apples and Strawberries Breakfast Mix

Preparation time: 10 minutes
Cooking time: 6 hours
Servings: 2

Ingredients:
- 1 cup water
- 6 ounces applesauce, unsweetened
- 3 tablespoons splenda
- ½ tablespoon cinnamon powder
- 3 ounces carrots, shredded
- 2 strawberries
- 1 tablespoon cardamom

Directions:
In your Crockpot, mix carrots with applesauce, splenda, cinnamon, strawberries and cardamom, stir, cover, cook on Low for 6 hours, divide between bowls and serve for breakfast.
Enjoy!

Nutrition: calories 139, fat 2, fiber 3, carbs 8, protein 4

Cauliflower and Mushroom Bowls

Preparation time: 10 minutes
Cooking time: 3 hours
Servings: 6

Ingredients:
- 1 cup cauliflower rice
- 6 green onions, chopped
- 3 tablespoons ghee, melted
- 2 garlic cloves, minced
- ½ pound Portobello mushrooms, sliced
- 2 cups warm water
- A pinch of salt and black pepper

Directions:
In your Crockpot, mix cauliflower rice with green onions, melted ghee, garlic, mushrooms, water, salt and pepper, stir well, cover, cook on Low for 3 hours, divide between bowls and serve for breakfast.
Enjoy!

Nutrition: calories 200, fat 5, fiber 3, carbs 7, protein 4

Turkey, Cranberries and Cauliflower Bowls

Preparation time: 10 minutes
Cooking time: 2 hours and 30 minutes
Servings: 12

Ingredients:
- ½ cup avocado oil
- 1 pound boiled turkey fillet, ground
- ½ pound mushrooms, sliced
- 6 celery ribs, chopped
- 2 yellow onions, chopped
- 2 garlic cloves, minced
- 1 tablespoon sage, chopped
- 1/3 cup cranberries, dried
- ½ cup cauliflower florets, chopped
- ½ cup veggie stock

Directions:
Heat up a pan with the oil over medium- high heat, add turkey meat, stir, brown for a couple of minutes and transfer to your Crockpot. Add mushrooms, celery, onion, garlic, sage, cranberries, cauliflower and stock, stir, cover and cook on High for 2 hours and 30 minutes. Divide between bowls and serve for breakfast.
Enjoy!

Nutrition: calories 200, fat 3, fiber 6, carbs 9, protein 4

Main Dish Recipes

Delicious Pork Chili

Preparation time: 10 minutes
Cooking time: 10 hours
Servings: 6

Ingredients:
- 3 garlic cloves, minced
- 2 pounds pork roast
- 2 tablespoons garlic powder
- 3 tablespoons smoked paprika
- ½ cup tomato passata
- 2 tablespoons chili powder
- 4 teaspoons cayenne pepper
- 1 tablespoon cumin, ground
- 1 tablespoon red pepper flakes
- A pinch of salt and black pepper
- 1 red bell pepper, chopped
- 2 yellow onions, chopped
- 1 yellow bell pepper, chopped
- 28 ounces canned tomatoes, chopped
- 14 ounces tomato sauce

Directions:
In your Crockpot, mix pork roast with garlic, tomato passata, paprika, chili powder, garlic powder, cumin, salt, pepper, cayenne, pepper flakes, red and yellow bell pepper, onion, tomatoes and tomato sauce, stir, cover and cook on Low for 10 hours. Shred meat, mix with the rest of the Ingredients one more time, divide between bowls and serve.
Enjoy!

Nutrition: calories 261, fat 7, fiber 4, carbs 8, protein 18

Spiced Pork Ribs

Preparation time: 10 minutes
Cooking time: 8 hours
Servings: 4

Ingredients:
- 4 pounds baby back pork ribs
- 2 teaspoons Chinese five spice powder
- A pinch of salt and black pepper
- ½ teaspoon garlic powder
- 1 jalapeno, roughly chopped
- 2 tablespoons coconut aminos
- 2 tablespoons white vinegar
- 1 tablespoon fresh tomato puree

Directions:
In your Crockpot, mix ribs with salt, pepper, Chinese five spice, garlic powder, aminos, jalapeno, vinegar and fresh tomato puree, toss well, cover and cook on Low for 8 hours. Divide ribs between plates and serve.
Enjoy!

Nutrition: calories 312, fat 7, fiber 7, carbs 8, protein 18

Delicious Pork Stew

Preparation time: 10 minutes
Cooking time: 6 hours
Servings: 4

Ingredients:
- 2 tablespoons coconut oil, melted
- 1 garlic clove, minced
- 1 yellow onion, chopped
- 2 pounds pork loin, cut into medium cubes
- A pinch of salt and black pepper
- 2 tablespoons dried mustard
- 2 tablespoons oregano, dried
- ½ teaspoon nutmeg, ground
- 1 pound oyster mushrooms
- 2 tablespoons white vinegar
- 1 and ½ cups veggie stock
- ¼ cup coconut milk
- 3 tablespoons capers

Directions:
In your Crockpot, mix oil with garlic, onion, pork cubes, salt, pepper, mustard, oregano, nutmeg, mushrooms, vinegar and stock, stir, cover and cook on Low for 5 hours. Add coconut milk and capers, toss, cover and cook on Low for 1 more hour. Divide between bowls and serve.
Enjoy!

Nutrition: calories 345, fat 7, fiber 5, carbs 14, protein 32

Simple Kalua Pork

Preparation time: 10 minutes
Cooking time: 12hours
Servings: 4

Ingredients:
- 3 pounds pork shoulder
- 1 tablespoon liquid smoke
- 3 tablespoons pink salt

Directions:
In your Crockpot, mix pork shoulder with smoke and salt, rub well, cover and cook on Low for 12hours. Slice pork, divide between plates and serve.
Enjoy!

Nutrition: calories 352, fat 8, fiber 4, carbs 10, protein 27

Tasty Pork Shanks

Preparation time: 10 minutes
Cooking time: 5 hours and 16 minutes
Servings: 4

Ingredients:
- 3 pounds pork shanks
- 1 and ½ tablespoons avocado oil
- ½ cups onion, chopped
- 1 cup butternut squash, chopped
- 4 garlic cloves, minced
- 1 tablespoon oregano, chopped
- 3 cups mushrooms, sliced
- 2 teaspoons thyme, chopped
- 2 tablespoons basil, chopped
- Zest and juice of 1 lemon
- A pinch of salt and black pepper
- 1 cup pumpkin puree
- 1 cup chicken stock

Directions:
Heat up a pan with ½ tablespoons oil over medium- high heat, add pork shanks, brown them for 8 minutes on each side and transfer them to your Crockpot. Add the rest of the oil, onion, squash, garlic, oregano, mushrooms, thyme, basil, lemon zest and juice, salt, pepper, pumpkin puree and stock, toss, cover and cook on High for 5 hours. Divide everything between plates and serve.
Enjoy!

Nutrition: calories 372, fat 7, fiber 5, carbs 12, protein 37

Simple Bacon and Collard Greens

Preparation time: 10 minutes
Cooking time: 5 hours
Servings: 4

Ingredients:
- ½ tablespoon coconut oil
- 6 bacon slices
- 1 yellow onion, chopped
- 4 garlic cloves, minced
- 1 pound collard greens, roughly chopped
- 2 cups chicken stock
- 2 tablespoons cider vinegar

Directions:
Heat up a pan over medium- high heat, add bacon, cook until it's crispy and transfer to your Crockpot. Heat up the same pan with the oil over medium heat, add garlic and collard greens, toss and cook them for a couple of minutes as well. Add greens to your Crockpot, also add onion, vinegar and stock, toss, cover and cook on Low for 5 hours. Divide between plates and serve.
Enjoy!

Nutrition: calories 273, fat 6, fiber 7, carbs 10, protein 17

Simple Pork and Cauliflower Rice

Preparation time: 10 minutes
Cooking time: 6 hours and 10 minutes
Servings: 4

Ingredients:
- 3 pounds pork roast
- 4 bacon slices, chopped
- A pinch of salt and black pepper
- 6 garlic cloves, minced
- 2 tablespoons liquid smoke
- 3 cups cauliflower, riced
- 2 tablespoons chicken stock
- ¼ teaspoon garlic powder
- A pinch of salt

For the cauliflower rice:

Directions:
In your Crockpot, mix pork with bacon, salt, pepper, garlic and smoke, toss well, cover and cook on High for 6 hours. During the last 10 minutes, heat up a pan over medium heat, add cauliflower, stock, salt and garlic powder, stir, cook for 10 minutes, transfer to your blender and pulse a bit. Slice pork and divide it between plates and serve with cauliflower rice on the side.
Enjoy!

Nutrition: calories 362, fat 8, fiber 8, carbs 10, protein 26

Chili Verde

Preparation time: 10 minutes
Cooking time: 8 hours
Servings: 4

Ingredients:
- 2 pounds pork stew meat, chopped
- 3 tablespoons cilantro, chopped
- 2 tablespoons olive oil
- 1 and ½ cups fresh tomato puree
- 2 tbsp chili powder
- 5 garlic cloves, minced
- A pinch of salt and black pepper

Directions:
In your Crockpot, mix pork meat with oil, tomato puree, garlic, salt, pepper and 2 tablespoons cilantro, toss, cover and cook on Low for 8 hours. Add the rest of the cilantro, toss, divide between bowls and serve.
Enjoy!

Nutrition: calories 292, fat 6, fiber 7, carbs 12, protein 22

Tender Pork Loin

Preparation time: 10 minutes
Cooking time: 12hours
Servings: 6

Ingredients:
- 1 yellow onion, cut into wedges
- 3 pounds pork loin
- 1 tablespoon sweet paprika
- 3 cups chicken stock
- A pinch of salt and black pepper

Directions:
In your Crockpot, mix pork loin with onions, paprika, stock, salt and pepper, cover and cook on Low for 12hours. Slice pork, divide it and onions between plates, drizzle cooking juices all over and serve.
Enjoy!

Nutrition: calories 322, fat 6, fiber 6, carbs 9, protein 22

Corned Beef Brisket

Preparation time: 10 minutes
Cooking time: 6 hours and 30 minutes
Servings: 4

Ingredients:
- 2 and ½ pounds beef brisket
- 1 yellow onion, chopped
- 1 celery stalk, roughly chopped
- 1 cup chicken stock
- 1 tablespoon avocado oil
- 1 green cabbage head, cut into medium wedges
- A pinch of salt and black pepper

For the cabbage:

Directions:
In your Crockpot, mix beef with onion, celery, and stock, toss, cover and cook on Low for 6 hours. Meanwhile, spread cabbage wedges on a lined baking sheet, season with salt and pepper, drizzle the oil, toss and bake In the oven at 360 degrees F for 30 minutes. Divide beef brisket between plates, add roasted cabbage on the side and serve.
Enjoy!

Nutrition: calories 251, fat 6, fiber 7, carbs 12, protein 6

Simple Beef Stew

Preparation time: 10 minutes
Cooking time: 4 hours and 30 minutes
Servings: 6

Ingredients:
- 2 pounds beef stew meat, cubed
- 1 teaspoon garlic powder
- A pinch of salt and black pepper
- 1 teaspoon onion powder
- 1 teaspoon thyme, dried
- 2 teaspoons sweet paprika
- 1 yellow onion, sliced
- 8 ounces white mushrooms, sliced
- 1/3 cup coconut cream
- 2 teaspoons red vinegar

Directions:
In your Crockpot, mix beef with garlic powder, salt, pepper, onion powder, thyme and paprika and rub well. Add onion, mushrooms, cream and vinegar, toss a bit, cover and cook on Low for 4 hours and 30 minutes. Divide between bowls and serve.
Enjoy!

Nutrition: calories 322, fat 5, fiber 7, carbs 9, protein 16

Spicy Curry

Preparation time: 10 minutes
Cooking time: 5 hours
Servings: 4

Ingredients:
- 2 and ½ pound beef chuck
- 4 garlic cloves, minced
- 1 red onion, chopped
- 1 Inch ginger piece, grated
- 2 tablespoons curry powder
- 2 cups coconut milk
- 2 tablespoons chili sauce
- A pinch of salt and black pepper

Directions:
In your Crockpot, mix beef chuck with curry powder, chili sauce, salt and pepper and rub well. In your food processor, mix onion with garlic, ginger and coconut milk, pulse well and add over beef mix. Cover pot, cook on Low for 5 hours, stir curry one more time, divide between bowls and serve.
Enjoy!

Nutrition: calories 352, fat 6, fiber 7, carbs 9, protein 18

Beef and Cabbage Stew

Preparation time: 10 minutes
Cooking time: 7 hours
Servings: 5

Ingredients:
- 4 oz bacon, cut into medium strips
- 2 red onions, chopped
- 3 pounds beef chuck roast, cut into medium cubes
- A pinch of salt and black pepper
- 1 garlic clove, crushed
- 1 Savoy cabbage, roughly chopped
- 1 thyme spring
- 1 cup beef stock

Directions:
Arrange bacon on the bottom of your Crockpot. Add onion, garlic, roast pieces, cabbage, thyme, salt, pepper and stock, cover pot and cook on Low for 7 hours. Divide between bowls and serve.
Enjoy!

Nutrition: calories 261, fat 7, fiber 6, carbs 8, protein 26

Beef and Veggie Stew

Preparation time: 10 minutes
Cooking time: 6 hours
Servings: 4

Ingredients:
- 1 pound beef meat, cubed
- 1 yellow onion, chopped
- 6 ounces fresh tomato puree
- 2 garlic cloves, minced
- 1 tablespoon thyme, chopped
- 5 oz butternut squash, chopped
- 3 celery stalks, chopped
- 2 bay leaves
- 2 tablespoons parsley, chopped
- 2 tablespoons white vinegar
- 1 tablespoon arrowroot powder
- A pinch of salt and black pepper

Directions:
In your Crockpot, mix beef with onion, fresh tomato puree, garlic, thyme, squash, celery, bay leaves, parsley, vinegar, arrowroot powder, salt and pepper, cover and cook on Low for 6 hours. Divide between bowls and serve.
Enjoy!

Nutrition: calories 300, fat 4, fiber 7, carbs 9, protein 22

Red Curry

Preparation time: 10 minutes
Cooking time: 8 hours
Servings: 4

Ingredients:
- 2 tablespoons coconut oil
- 2 tablespoons red curry paste
- 1 and ½ pounds beef stew meat, cubed
- 3 eggplants, cut into medium chunks
- 10 ounces coconut milk
- 1 teaspoon splenda
- 4 kaffir lime leaves

Directions:
In your Crockpot, mix oil with curry paste, beef stew meat, eggplants, coconut milk, splenda, and lime leaves, toss, cover and cook on Low for 8 hours. Divide between bowls and serve.
Enjoy!

Nutrition: calories 281, fat 7, fiber 6, carbs 8, protein 22

Tasty Meatballs

Preparation time: 10 minutes
Cooking time: 4 hours
Servings: 4

Ingredients:
- 3 pounds beef, ground
- ¼ cup spinach, chopped
- 1 teaspoon garlic powder
- 2 tablespoons onion, chopped
- A drizzle of olive oil
- A pinch of salt and black pepper
- 20 ounces tomato sauce

Directions:
In a bowl, mix beef with spinach, garlic powder, onion, salt and pepper, stir well and shape medium meatballs. Heat up a pan with the oil over medium-high heat, add meatballs, brown them on all sides, transfer to your Crockpot, cover them with the sauce and cook on Low for 4 hours. Divide meatballs and sauce between plates and serve.
Enjoy!

Nutrition: calories 322, fat 5, fiber 4, carbs 12, protein 22

Simple Shredded Beef

Preparation time : 10 minutes
Cooking time : 5 hours and 10 minutes
Servings: 4

Ingredients:
- 3 and ½ pounds beef roast
- ¼ cup veggie stock
- A pinch of salt and black pepper
- ½ teaspoon cumin, ground
- ½ tablespoon oregano, dried
- ¼ teaspoon ancho chili pepper
- A pinch of cinnamon powder
- ¼ teaspoon smoked paprika
- ½ teaspoon garlic powder
- 2 tablespoon fresh tomato puree
- 1 small yellow onion, chopped
- 1 jalapeno, chopped
- 3 garlic cloves, minced
- 1 cup fresh tomato puree

Directions:
In your Crockpot, mix beef roast with veggie stock, salt, pepper, cumin, oregano, chili pepper, cinnamon, paprika and garlic powder, toss well, cover and cook on Low for 5 hours. Shred meat, divide between plates and transfer 1 cup of cooking juices to a pan. Heat up cooking juices over medium- high heat, add onion, jalapeno, garlic, tomato puree, stir, simmer for 5 minutes and drizzle over shredded meat. Serve right away. Enjoy!

Nutrition: calories 391, fat 6, fiber 7, carbs 8, protein 27

American Beef Brisket

Preparation time: 10 minutes
Cooking time: 8 hours
Servings: 6

Ingredients:
- 3 pounds beef brisket
- A pinch of salt and black pepper
- 1 teaspoon fennel seeds
- 1 teaspoon cloves
- ½ teaspoon peppercorns
- 1 teaspoon cumin powder
- 1 teaspoon cardamom powder
- 3 tablespoons fresh tomato puree
- ½ teaspoon cinnamon powder
- 1 sweet onion, chopped
- 3 cups beef stock
- ¼ cup coconut vinegar

Directions:
In your Crockpot, mix beef brisket with salt, pepper, fennel, cloves, peppercorns, cumin, cardamom, cinnamon and fresh tomato puree and rub well. Add onion, stock and vinegar, toss, cover and cook on Low for 8 hours. Divide beef brisket and cooking juices between plates and serve.
Enjoy!

Nutrition: calories 392, fat 7, fiber 8, carbs 12, protein 28

Mexican Beef Stew

Preparation time: 10 minutes
Cooking time: 8 hours
Servings: 4

Ingredients:
- 1 pound beef stew meat, cubed
- 3 tomatoes, roughly chopped
- 1 red onion, chopped
- 1 garlic clove, minced
- 5 ounces canned green chilies, chopped
- 2 teaspoons chili powder
- 1 teaspoon cumin powder
- 1 teaspoon oregano, dried
- 2 cups water
- 2 cups beef stock
- A pinch of salt and black pepper

Directions:
Put meat In your Crockpot. Add tomatoes, onion, garlic, chilies, chili powder, cumin powder, oregano, water, stock, salt and pepper, cover and cook on Low for 8 hours. Divide between bowls and serve. Enjoy!

Nutrition: calories 328, fat 6, fiber 8, carbs 12, protein 28

Indian Beef Mix

Preparation time: 10 minutes
Cooking time: 5 hours
Servings: 4

Ingredients:
- 2 and ½ pounds beef roast
- 2 tablespoons coconut oil, melted
- 2 red onions, chopped
- 1 teaspoon black mustard seeds
- 25 curry leaves
- 2 tablespoons lemon juice
- 2 tablespoons garlic, minced
- 1 Inch ginger, grated
- 1 Serrano pepper, chopped
- 1 tablespoons coriander powder
- 2 teaspoons chili powder
- 1 teaspoon turmeric powder
- ½ teaspoon black peppercorns, ground
- ¼ cup coconut, unsweetened and shredded

Directions:
In your Crockpot, mix onions with salt, pepper, oil and mustard seeds, stir, cover and cook on High for 1 hour. Add beef roast, curry leaves, lemon juice, garlic, ginger, Serrano pepper, coriander, chili powder, turmeric powder and black peppercorns, toss a bit, cover and cook on High for 3 hours more. Add coconut, toss, cover and cook on High for 1 more hour. Divide between bowls and serve. Enjoy!

Nutrition: calories 300, fat 4, fiber 6, carbs 9, protein 22

Beef Tongue Mix

Preparation time: 10 minutes
Cooking time: 6 hours and 30 minutes
Servings: 4

Ingredients:
- 3 pounds beef tongue, sliced
- 2 jalapeno peppers, chopped
- 1 yellow onion, cut into wedges
- 1 red bell pepper, chopped
- 1 yellow bell pepper, chopped
- 5 garlic cloves, minced
- A pinch of salt and black pepper
- 2 tablespoons cayenne pepper
- 7 ounces fresh tomato puree
- 2 cups chicken stock
- 1 tablespoon olive oil
- 1 bunch green onions, chopped

Directions:
In your Crockpot, mix beef tongue with jalapenos, onion, red bell pepper, yellow bell pepper, garlic, salt, pepper, cayenne pepper, fresh tomato puree, stock, oil and green onions, toss, cover and cook on High for 6 hours. Divide tongue between plates and serve.
Enjoy!

Nutrition: calories 251, fat 6, fiber 3, carbs 7, protein 4

Ground Beef Soup

Preparation time: 10 minutes
Cooking time: 6 hours
Servings: 4

Ingredients:
- 1 pound beef, ground
- 2 zucchinis, chopped
- 3 oz butternut squash, chopped
- 1 yellow onion, chopped
- 1 celery stalk, chopped
- ½ cup veggie stock
- 3 cups water
- A pinch of salt and black pepper
- 29 ounces canned tomatoes, chopped
- 1 tablespoon garlic, minced
- ½ teaspoon oregano, dried
- ½ teaspoon basil, dried

Directions:
Heat up a pan over medium-high heat, add meat, brown on all sides and transfer to your Crockpot. Add water, zucchinis, squash, onion, celery, stock, salt, pepper, tomatoes, garlic, oregano and basil, stir, cover and cook on Low for 6 hours. Ladle Into bowls and serve.
Enjoy!

Nutrition: calories 271, fat 6, fiber 7, carbs 8, protein 12

Chicken Drumsticks

Preparation time: 10 minutes
Cooking time: 5 hours
Servings: 4

Ingredients:
- 10 chicken drumsticks, skinless
- 1 Inch ginger, grated
- 1 lemongrass stalk, trimmed and roughly chopped
- 5 garlic cloves minced
- 1 cup coconut milk
- 3 tablespoons coconut aminos
- 1 teaspoon five spice
- 1 yellow onion, chopped
- A pinch of salt and black pepper
- ¼ cup scallions, chopped

Directions:
In your Crockpot, mix drumsticks with ginger, lemongrass, garlic, coconut milk, aminos, five spice, onion, scallions, salt and pepper, toss, cover and cook on Low for 5 hours. Divide chicken and sauce between plates and serve right away.
Enjoy!

Nutrition: calories 210, fat 2, fiber 7, carbs 9, protein 16

Special Chicken Soup

Preparation time: 10 minutes
Cooking time: 8 hours
Servings: 10

Ingredients:
- 1 whole chicken, cut into medium pieces
- 20 basil leaves
- 1 lemongrass stalk, roughly chopped
- 4 ginger, slices
- Juice of 1 lime
- A pinch of salt and black pepper
- Water to cover

Directions:
In your Crockpot, mix chicken with basil, lemongrass, ginger, lime juice, salt, pepper and enough water to cover the meat, cover pot and cook on Low for 8 hours. Add more salt, stir, divide between bowls and serve.
Enjoy!

Nutrition: calories 211, fat 5, fiber 4, carbs 7, protein 12

Delicious Slow Cooked Chicken

Preparation time: 10 minutes
Cooking time: 5 hours
Servings: 4

Ingredients:
- 5 chicken drumsticks
- A pinch of salt and black pepper
- 1 teaspoon cayenne pepper
- 4 teaspoons sweet paprika
- 2 teaspoons onion powder
- 2 teaspoons thyme, dried
- 2 teaspoons garlic powder

Directions:
In a bowl, mix cayenne with salt, pepper, paprika, onion powder, thyme and garlic powder and stir. Rub chicken with this spice mix, put them In your Crockpot, cover and cook on Low for 5 hours. Discard bones and serve chicken with a side salad.
Enjoy!

Nutrition: calories 281, fat 4, fiber 6, carbs 7, protein 12

Delicious Bacon Chicken

Preparation time: 10 minutes
Cooking time: 8 hours
Servings: 4

Ingredients:
- 10 bacon slices
- 5 chicken breasts
- 2 tablespoons thyme, dried
- 1 teaspoon oregano, dried
- 1 tablespoon rosemary, dried
- 4 tablespoons olive oil
- A pinch of salt and black pepper

Directions:
In your Crockpot, mix bacon with chicken, thyme, oregano, rosemary, salt ,pepper and half of the oil, toss, cover and cook on Low for 8 hours. Add the rest of the oil, toss, divide chicken and bacon mix between plates and serve.
Enjoy!

Nutrition: calories 271, fat 7, fiber 4, carbs 7, protein 15

Chicken Curry

Preparation time: 10 minutes
Cooking time: 5 hours
Servings: 4

Ingredients:
- 3 pounds chicken thighs, skinless and boneless
- 3 tablespoons green curry paste
- 2 cups coconut milk

Directions:
In your Crockpot, mix chicken thighs with green curry paste and coconut milk, toss well, cover and cook n Low for 5 hours. Divide between bowls and serve right away.
Enjoy!

Nutrition: calories 211, fat 5, fiber 6, carbs 8, protein 12

Yellow Chicken Curry

Preparation time: 10 minutes
Cooking time: 6 hours
Servings: 4

Ingredients:
- 1 and ½ pounds chicken thighs, skinless, boneless and cut into medium chunks
- ½ cup butternut squash, chopped
- 1 cup broccoli florets
- 1 cup tomatoes, chopped
- 1 cup red bell pepper, chopped
- 14 ounces coconut milk
- 1 cup tomato sauce
- 1 teaspoon cumin, ground
- 2 teaspoons garlic powder
- 2 teaspoons ginger, grated
- 2 teaspoons coriander, ground
- 1 teaspoon cinnamon powder
- 1 cup water

Directions:
In your Crockpot, mix chicken thighs with squash, broccoli, tomatoes, red bell pepper, coconut milk, tomato sauce, cumin, garlic powder, ginger, coriander, cinnamon and water, cover and cook on Low for 6 hours. Divide between bowls and serve.
Enjoy!

Nutrition: calories 251, fat 6, fiber 6, carbs 12, protein 26

Delicious Shrimp

Preparation time: 10 minutes
Cooking time: 3 hours and 15 minutes
Servings: 4

Ingredients:
- 1 teaspoon avocado oil
- 1 pound shrimp, shelled
- A pinch of salt and black pepper
- 1 yellow onion, chopped
- 3 garlic cloves, minced
- 1 teaspoon red pepper flakes
- 15 ounces canned roasted tomatoes, chopped
- 1 tablespoon parsley, chopped

Directions:
Heat up a pan with the oil over medium- high heat, add garlic, onion and pepper flakes, stir, cook for 5 minutes and transfer to your Crockpot. Add tomatoes, salt, pepper and parsley to the pot as well, cover and cook on Low for 2 hours. Add shrimp, toss, cover and cook on High for 15 minutes. Divide shrimp mix between plates and serve.
Enjoy!

Nutrition: calories 251, fat 4, fiber 6, carbs 8, protein 12

Garlic Shrimp

Preparation time: 10 minutes
Cooking time: 50 minutes
Servings: 4

Ingredients:
- 2 pounds shrimp, peeled and deveined
- 1 tablespoons parsley, chopped
- A pinch of salt and black pepper
- ¼ teaspoon red pepper flakes, crushed
- 1 teaspoon smoked paprika
- 6 garlic cloves, minced
- ¾ cup olive oil

Directions:
In your Crockpot, mix oil, garlic, paprika, salt, pepper and red pepper flakes, stir, cover and cook on High for 30 minutes. Add shrimp and parsley, cover and cook on High for 10 minutes more. Stir again, cover pot again and cook on High for another 10 minutes. Divide between plates and serve.
Enjoy!

Nutrition: calories 200, fat 3, fiber 6, carbs 8, protein 11

Shrimp and Squash Mix

Preparation time: 10 minutes
Cooking time: 2 hours
Servings: 4

Ingredients:
- 1 pound spaghetti squash, peeled, halved and cubed
- 1 yellow onion, chopped
- 1 pound shrimp, deveined and peeled
- 2 and ½ teaspoons lemon- garlic seasoning
- 1 tablespoon olive oil
- 32 ounces chicken stock

Directions:
In your Crockpot, mix stock with lemon garlic seasoning, oil and onion and stir. Add squash, cover and cook on High for 2 hours. Add shrimp, cover and cook on High for 20 minutes. Divide between bowls and serve.
Enjoy!

Nutrition: calories 200, fat 3, fiber 4, carbs 7, protein 11

Simple Oxtail Stew

Preparation time: 10 minutes
Cooking time: 10 hours and 30 minutes
Servings: 4

Ingredients:
- 4 pounds oxtail, cut into medium segments
- 28 ounces canned tomatoes, chopped
- 2 cups water
- 4 teaspoons smoked paprika
- 10 garlic cloves, minced
- 2 tablespoons Italian seasoning
- A pinch of chili powder
- A pinch of salt and black pepper

Directions:
In your Crockpot, mix oxtail with the water, cover and cook on Low for 10 hours. Add garlic, tomatoes, paprika, Italian seasoning, salt, pepper and chili powder, toss, cover and cook on High for 30 minutes more. Divide stew Into bowls and serve.
Enjoy!

Nutrition: calories 261, fat 3, fiber 6, carbs 8, protein 11

Lamb Leg

Preparation time: 10 minutes
Cooking time: 10 hours
Servings: 4

Ingredients:
- 4 pounds lamb leg
- A pinch of salt and black pepper
- 1 and ½ teaspoon thyme, dried
- 2 garlic cloves, minced
- 1 tablespoon olive oil
- 3 cups beef stock
- 3 tablespoons almond flour

Directions:
Put lamb leg In your Crockpot, add salt, pepper, thyme, garlic, oil and stock, stir, cover and cook on Low for 10 hours. Transfer lamb leg to a cutting board, slice and divide between plates. Transfer 2 cups cooking juices to a pot, add almond flour, stir, heat up over medium heat, cook for 1-2 minutes, drizzle over lamb and serve. Enjoy!

Nutrition: calories 433, fat 12, fiber 4, carbs 6, protein 28

Rabbit Stew

Preparation time: 10 minutes
Cooking time: 6 hours
Servings: 4

Ingredients:
- 1 rabbit, legs removed
- 1 pound boiled turkey fillet, sliced
- 4 oz butternut squash, roughly chopped
- 1 yellow onion, chopped
- 2 quarts chicken stock
- ¼ teaspoon red pepper flakes
- 7 ounces mushrooms, sliced
- ¼ teaspoon sweet paprika
- 1 tablespoon coconut oil, melted
- A pinch of salt and black pepper
- A pinch of cayenne

Directions:
Put the oil In your Crockpot and add rabbit. Add turkey fillet, squash, onion, pepper flakes, stock, mushrooms, paprika, salt, pepper and cayenne, toss, cover and cook on High for 6 hours. Carve rabbit, divide it and veggies Into bowls and serve.
Enjoy!

Nutrition: calories 521, fat 7, fiber 4, carbs 7, protein 38

Beef Roast Soup

Preparation time: 10 minutes
Cooking time: 7 hours
Servings: 4

Ingredients:
- 2 pounds beef roast
- 1 red onion, sliced
- 2 quarts beef stock
- 4 thyme springs
- ½ cup sherry vinegar
- 1 bay leaf
- A pinch of salt and black pepper
- 2 tablespoons olive oil

Directions:
In your Crockpot, mix beef roast with stock, bay leaf and thyme, cover, cook on High for 6 hours, transfer roast to a cutting board, cool it down, shred and transfer to a bowl. Heat up a large pot with the oil over medium- high heat, add onions, stir and cook them for 5 minutes. Add vinegar, stock from the Crockpot, salt, pepper and beef, stir and cook for 45 minutes. Divide beef soup Into bowls and serve.
Enjoy!

Nutrition: calories 632, fat 7, fiber 7, carbs 12, protein 37

Easy Lamb Curry

Preparation time: 10 minutes
Cooking time: 6 hours
Servings: 2

Ingredients:
- 3 tablespoons madras curry paste
- 1 yellow onion, sliced
- 10 ounces canned tomatoes, chopped
- 1 tablespoon ginger, grated
- 1 teaspoon cumin seeds
- 1 cinnamon stick
- 1 cup kale, chopped
- 2 lean lamb steaks, chopped

Directions:
In your Crockpot, mix lamb with curry paste, onion, tomatoes, ginger, cumin, cinnamon and kale, toss, cover and cook on Low for 6 hours. Discard cinnamon stick, stir curry, divide between bowls and serve.
Enjoy!

Nutrition: calories 261, fat 4, fiber 4, carbs 8, protein 12

Lamb Shoulder Mix

Preparation time: 10 minutes
Cooking time: 8 hours
Servings: 4

Ingredients:
- 1 and ½ pounds lamb shoulder joint
- 6 oz butternut squash, cut into medium chunks
- 10 ounces lamb stock
- A pinch of salt and black pepper
- A handful mint, chopped

Directions:
In your Crockpot, mix lamb with squash, stock, salt, pepper and mint, cover and cook on Low for 8 hours. Divide lamb and cooking juices between plates and serve.
Enjoy!

Nutrition: calories 281, fat 7, fiber 7, carbs 12, protein 6

Delicious Creamy Chicken

Preparation time: 10 minutes
Cooking time: 6 hours
Servings: 4

Ingredients:
- 1 and ½ pounds chicken thighs, boneless
- 2 teaspoons sweet paprika
- 1 tablespoon chili powder
- 1 teaspoon cumin, ground
- 1 teaspoon coriander, ground
- 1 teaspoon garlic powder
- A pinch of salt and white pepper
- A pinch of cayenne pepper
- 1 cup chicken stock
- 2 red bell peppers, chopped
- ¼ cup lime juice
- ½ cup coconut cream
- 2 tablespoons parsley, chopped

Directions:
In a bowl, mix chicken thighs with paprika, chili powder, cumin, coriander, garlic powder, salt, pepper and cayenne and rub well. Heat up a pan over medium- high heat, add chicken pieces, brown them for a few minutes on each side and transfer to your Crockpot. Add stock, lime juice and top with bell peppers, cover pot and cook on Low for 5 hours and 30 minutes. Add cream and parsley, toss a bit, cover and cook on Low for 30 minutes more. Divide between bowls and serve.
Enjoy!

Nutrition: calories 322, fat 6, fiber 7, carbs 8, protein 18

Creamy Salmon Soup

Preparation time: 10 minutes
Cooking time: 7 hours
Servings: 6

Ingredients:
- 2 tablespoons avocado oil
- 4 leeks, sliced
- 3 garlic cloves, minced
- 6 cups chicken stock
- 2 teaspoons thyme, dried
- 1 pounds salmon, skinless, boneless and cut into medium cubes
- 1 and ¼ cup coconut milk
- A pinch of salt and black pepper

Directions:
Heat up a pan with the oil over medium- high heat, add garlic and leeks, stir, brown for a few minutes and transfer to your Crockpot. Add stock, thyme, salt and pepper, cover and cook on Low for 3 hours. Add coconut milk and salmon, cover and cook on Low for 1 more hour. Ladle Into bowls and serve.
Enjoy!

Nutrition: calories 232, fat 4, fiber 7, carbs 9, protein 11

Shrimp Stew

Preparation time: 10 minutes
Cooking time: 7 hours and 30 minutes
Servings: 6

Ingredients:
- 1 pounds fried turkey meat, sliced
- 1 yellow onion, roughly chopped
- 2 celery stalks, chopped
- 2 garlic cloves, minced
- 1 green bell pepper, chopped
- 28 ounces canned tomatoes, chopped
- ¼ cup water
- A pinch of salt and black pepper
- A pinch of cayenne pepper
- 1 pound shrimp, deveined

Directions:
Put turkey, onion, bell pepper and celery In your Crockpot. Add water, tomatoes, salt, pepper and cayenne, cover and cook on Low for 7 hours. Add shrimp, cover and cook on High for 30 minutes. Divide stew Into bowls and serve.
Enjoy!

Nutrition: calories 321, fat 4, fiber 7, carbs 8, protein 4

Tasty Seafood Stew

Preparation time: 10 minutes
Cooking time: 4 hours
Servings: 6

Ingredients:
- 28 ounces canned tomatoes, crushed
- 3 garlic cloves, minced
- 4 cups veggie stock
- 1 yellow onion, chopped
- 1 teaspoon basil, dried
- 1 teaspoon thyme, dried
- 1 teaspoon cilantro, dried
- A pinch of salt and black pepper
- ¼ teaspoon red pepper flakes
- A pinch of cayenne pepper
- 2 pounds mixed deveined shrimp, scallops and crab legs

Directions:
In your Crockpot, mix tomatoes with cloves, stock, onion, basil, thyme, cilantro, salt, pepper, pepper flakes and cayenne, cover and cook on High for 3 hours. Add mixed seafood, cover and cook on High for 1 more hour. Divide between bowls and serve right away.
Enjoy!

Nutrition: calories 251, fat 4, fiber 6, carbs 8, protein 12

Seafood Chowder

Preparation time: 10 minutes
Cooking time: 8 hours and 30 minutes
Servings: 4

Ingredients:
- 2 cups water
- ½ fennel bulb, chopped
- 1 yellow onion, chopped
- 2 bay leaves
- 1 tablespoon thyme, dried
- 1 celery rib, chopped
- A pinch of salt and black pepper
- A pinch of cayenne pepper
- 1 cup seafood stock
- 1 cup coconut milk
- 1 pounds salmon fillets, cubed
- 5 sea scallops, halved
- 24 shrimp, peeled and deveined
- ¼ cup parsley, chopped

Directions:
In your Crockpot, mix water with fennel, onion, bay leaves, thyme, celery, stock, cayenne, salt and black pepper, cover and cook on Low for 8 hours. Add salmon, coconut milk, scallops, shrimp and parsley, cover, cook on Low for 30 minutes more, ladle chowder Into bowls and serve.
Enjoy!

Nutrition: calories 354, fat 10, fiber 2, carbs 7, protein 12

Maple Salmon with Broccoli and Cauliflower

Preparation time: 10 minutes
Cooking time: 3 hours
Servings: 2

Ingredients:
- 2 medium salmon fillets, boneless
- A pinch of sea salt and black pepper
- 2 tablespoons coconut aminos
- 2 tablespoons sugar-free maple syrup
- 16 ounces mixed broccoli and cauliflower florets
- 2 tablespoons lemon juice
- 1 teaspoon sesame seeds

Directions:
Put the cauliflower and broccoli florets In your Crockpot and top with salmon fillets. In a bowl, mix sugar-free maple syrup with aminos and lemon juice and whisk really well. Pour this over salmon fillets, season with salt and black pepper, sprinkle sesame seeds on top and cook on Low for 3 hours. Divide everything between plates and serve right away.
Enjoy!

Nutrition: calories 230, fat 4, fiber 2, carbs 7, protein 6

Italian Shrimp

Preparation time: 10 minutes
Cooking time: 1 hour and 30 minutes
Servings: 4

Ingredients:
- 2 tablespoons olive oil
- ¼ cup chicken stock
- 1 tablespoon garlic, minced
- 2 tablespoons parsley, chopped
- Juice of ½ lemon
- A pinch of salt and black pepper to the taste
- 1 pound shrimp, peeled and deveined

Directions:
Put the oil In your Crockpot, add stock, garlic, parsley, lemon juice, salt and pepper and whisk. Add shrimp, stir, cover and cook on High for 1 hour and 30 minutes. Divide between bowls and serve.
Enjoy!

Nutrition: calories 140, fat 4, fiber 3, carbs 9, protein 3

Thai Pompano with Leeks

Preparation time: 10 minutes
Cooking time: 1 hour
Servings: 4

Ingredients:
- 1 pompano
- 2 tablespoons coconut aminos
- ¼ cup olive oil
- ¼ cup veggie stock
- 1 small ginger piece, grated
- 6 garlic cloves, minced
- 2 tablespoons soy sauce
- 1 bunch leeks, chopped
- 1 bunch cilantro, chopped

Directions:
Put the oil In your Crockpot, add leeks and top with the fish. In a bowl, mix stock with ginger, garlic, soy sauce, cilantro and aminos, whisk well, add to the pot, cover and cook on High for 1 hour. Divide fish between plates and serve with the sauce drizzled on top.
Enjoy!

Nutrition: calories 300, fat 8, fiber 2, carbs 8, protein 6

Spicy Tuna Loin

Preparation time: 10 minutes
Cooking time: 4 hours and 10 minutes
Servings: 2

Ingredients:
- ½ pound tuna loin, cubed
- 1 garlic clove, minced
- 4 jalapeno peppers, chopped
- 1 cup olive oil
- 3 red chili peppers, chopped
- 2 teaspoons black peppercorns, ground
- A pinch of salt and black pepper to the taste

Directions:
Put the oil In your Crockpot, add chili peppers, jalapenos, peppercorns, salt, pepper and garlic, whisk, cover and cook on Low for 4 hours. Add tuna cubes, cook on High for 10 minutes more, divide between plates and serve.
Enjoy!

Nutrition: calories 200, fat 4, fiber 3, carbs 7, protein 4

Braised Squid

Preparation time: 10 minutes
Cooking time: 7 hours
Servings: 4

Ingredients:
- 1 pound squid, cleaned and cut into rings
- 1/2 cup stevia
- 1 small ginger piece, grated
- 1 garlic head, peeled and crushed
- 3 tablespoons coconut aminos
- 1/4 cup veggie stock
- 2 leeks stalks, chopped
- 2 bay leaves
- A pinch of salt and black pepper

Directions:
Put the squid In your Crockpot, add stevia, ginger, garlic, aminos, leeks, stock, black pepper and bay leaves, stir, cover and cook on Low for 8 hours. Divide between bowls and serve right away.
Enjoy!

Nutrition: calories 190, fat 2, fiber 4, carbs 7, protein 5

Salmon with Cilantro Sauce

Preparation time: 10 minutes
Cooking time: 2 hours and 30 minutes
Servings: 4

Ingredients:
- 2 garlic cloves, minced
- 4 salmon fillets, boneless
- ¾ cup cilantro, chopped
- 3 tablespoons lime juice
- 1 tablespoon olive oil
- A pinch of salt and black pepper to the taste

Directions:
Grease your Crockpot with the oil, place salmon fillets inside skin side down, add garlic, cilantro, lime juice, salt and pepper, cover and cook on Low for 2 hours and 30 minutes. Divide salmon fillets on plates, drizzle cilantro sauce from the Crockpot all over and serve.
Enjoy!

Nutrition: calories 180, fat 3, fiber 2, carbs 4, protein 8

Steamed Salmon

Preparation time: 10 minutes
Cooking time: 2 hours
Servings: 2

Ingredients:
- 1 medium salmon fillets
- A pinch of nutmeg, ground
- A pinch of cloves, ground
- A pinch of ginger powder
- A pinch of sea salt
- 2 teaspoons stevia
- 1 teaspoon onion powder
- ¼ teaspoon chipotle chili powder
- ½ teaspoon cayenne pepper
- A pinch of salt and black pepper
- ½ teaspoon cinnamon powder
- ½ teaspoon thyme, dried

Directions:
In a bowl, mix salmon fillets with nutmeg, cloves, ginger, salt, stevia, onion powder, chili powder, cayenne black pepper, cinnamon and thyme, rub, divide fish on 2 tin foil pieces, wrap, place In your Crockpot, cover and cook on Low for 2 hours. Unwrap fish, divide between plates and serve with a side salad.
Enjoy!

Nutrition: calories 220, fat 4, fiber 2, carbs 7, protein 4

Creamy Clams

Preparation time: 10 minutes
Cooking time: 6 hours
Servings: 4

Ingredients:
- 21 ounces canned clams, chopped
- 1/3 cup coconut milk
- 4 eggs, whisked
- 2 tablespoons olive oil
- 1/3 cup green bell pepper, chopped
- ½ cup yellow onion, chopped
- Black pepper to the taste
- A pinch of sea salt

Directions:
Put clams In your Crockpot. In a bowl, mix milk, eggs, oil, onion, bell pepper, a pinch of salt and black pepper, whisk and add over clams. Stir, cover, cook on Low for 6 hours, divide between bowls and serve.
Enjoy!

Nutrition: calories 190, fat 4, fiber 2, carbs 6, protein 7

Side Dishes

Mexican Veggie Mix

Preparation time: 10 minutes
Cooking time: 2 hours
Servings: 4

Ingredients:
- 1 cup butternut squash, shredded
- 1 celery stalk, chopped
- ½ green cabbage head, shredded
- 2 zucchinis, chopped
- ½ sweet onion, chopped
- 4 tomatoes, chopped
- 2 tablespoons fresh tomato puree
- 5 garlic cloves, minced
- 2 jalapenos, chopped
- 1 cup cilantro, chopped
- 3 cups chicken stock
- 1 tablespoon cumin, ground
- 1 tablespoon chili powder
- A drizzle of olive oil
- A pinch of salt and black pepper

Directions:
Grease your Crockpot with the oil and arrange squash, celery, cabbage, zucchinis, onion and tomatoes in the pot. Add fresh tomato puree, garlic, jalapenos, cilantro, stock, cumin, chili powder, salt and pepper, cover and cook on Low for 2 hours. Divide between plates and serve as a side dish.
Enjoy!

Nutrition: calories 211, fat 3, fiber 3, carbs 6, protein 8

Fresh Veggie Side Dish

Preparation time: 10 minutes
Cooking time: 3 hours
Servings: 4

Ingredients:
- 2 cups okra, sliced
- ½ cup red onion, roughly chopped
- 1 cup cherry tomatoes, halved
- 2 and ½ cups zucchini, sliced
- 2 cups red and yellow bell peppers, sliced
- 1 cup white mushrooms, sliced
- ½ cup olive oil
- ½ cup balsamic vinegar
- 2 tablespoons basil, chopped
- 1 tablespoon thyme, chopped

Directions:
In your Crockpot, mix okra with onion, tomatoes, zucchini, bell peppers, mushrooms, basil and thyme. In a bowl mix oil with vinegar, whisk well, add to the pot, cover and cook on High for 3 hours. Divide between plates and serve as a side dish.
Enjoy!

Nutrition: calories 233, fat 12, fiber 4, carbs 8, protein 4

Spinach and Squash Mix

Preparation time: 10 minutes
Cooking time: 4 hours
Servings: 6

Ingredients:
- 10 oz butternut squash, sliced
- 2 garlic cloves, minced
- 1 yellow onion, chopped
- A pinch of salt and black pepper
- ½ teaspoon oregano, dried
- 5 ounces baby spinach
- 2 and ½ cups veggie stock
- 2 teaspoons lemon peel, grated
- 3 tablespoons lemon juice
- 1 avocado, pitted, peeled and chopped
- ¾ cup goat cheese, crumbled

Directions:
In your Crockpot, mix onion, squash, garlic, salt, pepper, oregano and stock, stir, cover and cook on High for 4 hours. Add spinach, lemon juice and lemon peel, stir, leave aside for 5 minutes, divide between plates, sprinkle goat cheese and avocado on top and serve as a side dish.
Enjoy!

Nutrition: calories 219, fat 8, fiber 4, carbs 8, protein 17

Cauliflower and Broccoli Fresh Mix

Preparation time: 10 minutes
Cooking time: 3 hours
Servings: 10

Ingredients:
- 4 cups broccoli florets
- 4 cups cauliflower florets
- 14 ounces fresh tomato puree
- 1 yellow onion, chopped
- 1 teaspoon thyme, dried
- Salt and black pepper to the taste
- ½ cup almonds, sliced

Directions:
In your Crockpot, mix broccoli with cauliflower, fresh tomato puree, onion, thyme, salt and pepper, toss, cover and cook on High for 3 hours. Divide between plates and serve as a side dish with almonds sprinkled on top.
Enjoy!

Nutrition: calories 177, fat 12, fiber 2, carbs 7, protein 7

Special Cauliflower Rice Mix

Preparation time: 10 minutes
Cooking time: 6 hours
Servings: 12

Ingredients:
- 2 cups veggie stock
- 2 and ½ cups cauliflower rice
- 1 cup butternut squash, shredded
- 4 ounces mushrooms, sliced
- 2 tablespoons olive oil
- 2 teaspoons marjoram, dried and crushed
- Salt and black pepper to the taste
- 2/3 cup dried cherries
- 2/3 cup green onions, chopped

Directions:
In your Crockpot, mix stock with cauliflower rice, squash, mushrooms, oil, marjoram, salt, pepper, cherries and green onions, toss, cover and cook on Low for 6 hours. Divide between plates and serve as a side dish. Enjoy!

Nutrition: calories 169, fat 5, fiber 3, carbs 8, protein 5

Rustic Mashed Cauliflower

Preparation time: 10 minutes
Cooking time: 4 hours
Servings: 6

Ingredients:
- 6 garlic cloves, peeled
- 1 big cauliflower head, florets separated
- 1 bay leaf
- 1 cup coconut milk
- 3 cups veggie stock
- 1 tablespoons olive oil
- Salt and black pepper to the taste

Directions:
In your Crockpot, mix cauliflower with stock, bay leaf, garlic, salt and pepper, cover and cook on High for 4 hours. Drain cauliflower mix, return to your Crockpot and mash using a potato masher. Add oil and coconut milk, whisk well, divide between plates and serve as a side dish.
Enjoy!

Nutrition: calories 135, fat 5, fiber 1, carbs 7, protein 3

Squash and Parsnips Mix

Preparation time: 10 minutes
Cooking time: 4 hours
Servings: 10

Ingredients:
- 1 pound parsnips, cut into medium chunks
- 10 oz butternut squash, cut into medium chunks
- 2 tablespoons lemon peel, grated
- 1 cup veggie stock
- A pinch of salt and black pepper
- 3 tablespoons olive oil
- ¼ cup parsley, chopped

Directions:
In your Crockpot, mix parsnips with squash, lemon peel, stock, salt, pepper, oil and parsley, cover and cook on High for 4 hours. Divide between plates and serve as a side dish.
Enjoy!

Nutrition: calories 159, fat 4, fiber 4, carbs 6, protein 2

Summer Greenie Mix

Preparation time: 10 minutes
Cooking time: 3 hours and 30 minutes
Servings: 10

Ingredients:
- 10 ounces spinach, torn
- 1 pound butternut squash, peeled and cubed
- 1 yellow onion, chopped
- 2 cups veggie stock
- ½ cup water
- A pinch of salt and black pepper
- 3 garlic cloves, minced

Directions:
In your Crockpot, mix squash with spinach, onion, stock, water, salt, pepper and garlic, toss, cover and cook on High for 3 hours and 30 minutes. Divide squash mix on plates and serve as a side dish.
Enjoy!

Nutrition: calories 196, fat 3, fiber 7, carbs 8, protein 7

Fall Veggie Mix

Preparation time: 10 minutes
Cooking time: 8 hours
Servings: 6

Ingredients:
- 2 tablespoons olive oil
- 2 tablespoons rosemary, chopped
- A pinch of salt and black pepper
- 2 cups cherry tomatoes, halved
- 2 garlic cloves, minced
- 1 pound cauliflower, florets separated
- 6 oz acorn squash, peeled
- 28 ounces veggie stock
- 1 yellow onion, cut into medium wedges
- 4 cups baby spinach
- 8 ounces zucchini, sliced

Directions:
In your Crockpot, mix oil, rosemary, salt, pepper, cherry tomatoes, garlic, cauliflower, squash, onion, zucchini, spinach and stock, stir, cover and cook on Low for 8 hours. Divide everything between plates and serve as a side dish.
Enjoy!

Nutrition: calories 273, fat 7, fiber 5, carbs 8, protein 12

Eggplant and Kale Mix

Preparation time: 10 minutes
Cooking time: 2 hours
Servings: 6

Ingredients:
- 14 ounces canned roasted tomatoes and garlic
- 4 cups eggplant, cubed
- 1 yellow bell pepper, chopped
- 1 red onion, cut into medium wedges
- 4 cups kale leaves
- 2 tablespoons olive oil
- 1 teaspoon mustard
- 3 tablespoons red vinegar
- 1 garlic clove, minced
- A pinch of salt and black pepper
- ½ cup basil, chopped

Directions:
In your Crockpot, mix the eggplant cubes with tomatoes, bell pepper and onion, toss, cover and cook on High for 2 hours. Add kale, toss, cover Crockpot and leave aside for now. Meanwhile, in a bowl, mix oil with vinegar, mustard, garlic, salt and pepper and whisk well. Add this and basil over eggplant mix, toss, divide between plates and serve as a side dish.
Enjoy!

Nutrition: calories 251, fat 9, fiber 6, carbs 7, protein 8

Brussels Sprouts and Onions

Preparation time: 10 minutes
Cooking time: 3 hours
Servings: 10

Ingredients:
- 1/3 cup red onion, chopped
- 2 pounds Brussels sprouts, trimmed and halved
- A pinch of salt and black pepper
- ¼ cup apple juice
- 3 tablespoons olive oil
- ¼ cup sugar-free maple syrup
- 1 tablespoon thyme, chopped

Directions:
In your Crockpot, mix sprouts with onion, salt, pepper and apple juice, toss, cover and cook on Low for 3 hours. In a bowl, mix sugar-free maple syrup with oil and thyme, whisk really well, add over sprouts mix, toss, divide between plates and serve as a side dish.
Enjoy!

Nutrition: calories 100, fat 4, fiber 4, carbs 8, protein 3

Cabbage and Apples Side Dish

Preparation time: 10 minutes
Cooking time: 6 hours
Servings: 4

Ingredients:
- 1 onion, sliced
- 1 cabbage, shredded
- 2 apples, peeled, cored and roughly chopped
- A pinch of salt and black pepper
- 1 cup apple juice
- ½ cup chicken stock
- 3 tablespoons mustard
- 1 tablespoon coconut oil, melted

Directions:
Grease your Crockpot with the coconut oil and place apples, cabbage and onions Inside. In a bowl, mix stock with mustard, salt, black pepper and the apple juice, whisk well, add to Crockpot, cover and cook on Low for 6 hours. Divide between plates and serve right away as a side dish.
Enjoy!

Nutrition: calories 200, fat 4, fiber 2, carbs 8, protein 6

Simple Mushrooms Caps Side Dish

Preparation time: 10 minutes
Cooking time: 4 hours
Servings: 4

Ingredients:
- 2 bay leaves
- 4 garlic cloves, minced
- 14 ounces white mushroom caps
- ¼ teaspoon thyme dried
- ½ teaspoon basil, dried
- ½ teaspoon oregano, dried
- 1 cup veggie stock
- A pinch of salt and black pepper
- 2 tablespoons olive oil
- 2 tablespoons parsley, chopped

Directions:
Grease your Crockpot with the oil, add mushrooms, garlic, bay leaves, thyme, basil, oregano, black pepper and stock, cover and cook on Low for 4 hours. Divide between plates and serve with parsley sprinkled on top as a side dish.
Enjoy!

Nutrition: calories 122, fat 6, fiber 1, carbs 8, protein 5

Zucchini and Squash Side Dish

Preparation time: 10 minutes
Cooking time: 6 hours
Servings: 6

Ingredients:
- 2 cups zucchinis, sliced
- 1 teaspoon Italian seasoning
- Black pepper to the taste
- 2 cups butternut squash, peeled and cut into wedges
- 1 teaspoon garlic powder
- 2 tablespoons olive oil
- A pinch of salt and black pepper

Directions:
Grease your Crockpot with the oil, add zucchini, squash, Italian seasoning, black pepper, salt and garlic powder, toss well, cover and cook on Low for 6 hours. Divide between plates and serve as a side dish.
Enjoy!

Nutrition: calories 100, fat 2, fiber 4, carbs 8, protein 5

Cheesy Green Beans

Preparation time: 10 minutes
Cooking time: 3 hours and 30 minutes
Servings: 4

Ingredients:
- 2/3 cup parmesan, grated
- 1 egg
- 12 ounces green beans
- Salt and black pepper to the taste
- ½ teaspoon garlic powder
- ¼ teaspoon sweet paprika

Directions:
In a bowl, mix the egg with parmesan with salt, pepper, garlic powder and paprika and whisk. Put green beans In your Crockpot, add egg and parmesan mix over them, toss well, cover and cook on Low for 3 hours and 30 minutes. Divide between plates and serve as a side dish.
Enjoy!

Nutrition: calories 114, fat 5, fiber 6, carbs 8, protein 9

Herbed Mushrooms Mix

Preparation time: 10 minutes
Cooking time: 3 hours
Servings: 4

Ingredients:
- 12 ounces Portobello mushrooms, sliced
- Salt and black pepper to the taste
- ½ teaspoon basil, dried
- 2 tablespoons olive oil
- ½ teaspoon tarragon, dried
- ½ teaspoon rosemary, dried
- ½ teaspoon thyme, dried
- 2 tablespoons balsamic vinegar

Directions:
In a bowl, mix oil with vinegar, salt, pepper, rosemary, tarragon, basil and thyme and whisk well. Add mushroom slices, toss to coat well, transfer to your Crockpot, cover and cook on Low for 3 hours. Divide between plates and serve as a side dish.
Enjoy!

Nutrition: calories 80, fat 4, fiber 4, carbs 8, protein 4

Brussels Sprouts and Bacon

Preparation time: 10 minutes
Cooking time: 6 hours
Servings: 4

Ingredients:
- 8 bacon strips, chopped
- 1 pound Brussels sprouts, trimmed and halved
- Salt and black pepper to the taste
- A pinch of cumin, ground
- A pinch of red pepper, crushed
- 2 tablespoons olive oil

Directions:
In a bowl, mix Brussels sprouts with salt, pepper, cumin, red pepper and oil, toss to coat, transfer to your Crockpot, add bacon on top, cover and cook on Low for 6 hours. Divide between plates and serve as a side dish.
Enjoy!

Nutrition: calories 256, fat 12, fiber 6, carbs 8, protein 15

Creamy Spinach

Preparation time: 10 minutes
Cooking time: 3 hours
Servings: 2

Ingredients:
- 2 garlic cloves, minced
- 8 ounces spinach leaves
- A drizzle of olive oil
- Salt and black pepper to the taste
- 4 tablespoons coconut cream
- 2 tablespoons parmesan cheese, grated

Directions:
Grease your Crockpot with the oil, add garlic, spinach, salt, pepper and coconut cream, toss, cover and cook on Low for 3 hours. Add parmesan, toss until it melts, divide between plates and serve as a side dish.
Enjoy!

Nutrition: calories 133, fat 10, fiber 4, carbs 4, protein 2

Okra and Mint

Preparation time: 10 minutes
Cooking time: 3 hours
Servings: 4

Ingredients:
- 1 pound okra, sliced
- Salt and black pepper to the taste
- 1 tablespoon mint, chopped
- 2 teaspoons olive oil
- 2 tablespoons chicken stock
- 3 green onions, chopped
- 1 garlic clove, minced

Directions:
Grease your Crockpot with the oil, add okra, salt, pepper, mint, stock, garlic and green onions, toss, cover and cook on Low for 3 hours. Divide between plates and serve as a side dish.
Enjoy!

Nutrition: calories 70, fat 1, fiber 1, carbs 4, protein 6

Napa Cabbage Mix

Preparation time: 10 minutes
Cooking time: 2 hours
Servings: 6

Ingredients:
- 1 pound napa cabbage, chopped
- A pinch of salt and black pepper
- 4 oz butternut squash, julienned
- 2 tablespoons veggie stock
- ½ cup radish, sliced
- 3 garlic cloves, minced
- 3 green onion stalks, chopped
- 1 tablespoon coconut aminos
- 3 tablespoons chili flakes
- 1 tablespoon olive oil
- ½ Inch ginger, grated

Directions:
In your Crockpot, mix cabbage with salt, pepper, squash, stock, radish, garlic, green onions, aminos, chili flakes, oil and ginger, toss, cover and cook on High for 2 hours. Divide between plates and serve as a side dish.
Enjoy!

Nutrition: calories 100, fat 3, fiber 4, carbs 5, protein 2

Garlicky Swiss Chard

Preparation time: 10 minutes
Cooking time: 2 hours
Servings: 4

Ingredients:
- 2 tablespoons olive oil
- 3 tablespoons lemon juice
- ½ cup chicken stock
- 4 bacon slices, chopped
- 2 bunches Swiss chard, roughly torn
- ½ teaspoon garlic paste
- Salt and black pepper to the taste

Directions:
In your Crockpot, mix oil with chard, bacon, stock, lemon juice, garlic paste, salt and pepper, toss, cover and cook on High for 2 hours. Divide between plates and serve as a side dish.
Enjoy

Nutrition: calories 160, fat 7, fiber 3, carbs 6, protein 4

Mushroom and Arugula Mix

Preparation time: 10 minutes
Cooking time: 2 hours
Servings: 4

Ingredients:
- 2 tablespoons olive oil
- Salt and black pepper to the taste
- 1 pound cremini mushrooms, roughly chopped
- 4 tablespoons veggie stock
- 4 bunches arugula
- 8 slices prosciutto, chopped
- 2 tablespoons balsamic vinegar
- 8 sun dried tomatoes, chopped
- 1 tablespoon parsley, chopped

Directions:
In your Crockpot, mix mushrooms with oil, salt, pepper, stock, prosciutto, vinegar and tomatoes, toss, cover and cook on High for 2 hours. Add arugula and parsley, toss, leave aside for a few minutes, divide between plates and serve as a side dish.
Enjoy!

Nutrition: calories 200, fat 3, fiber 2, carbs 5, protein 6

Red Chard Mix

Preparation time: 10 minutes
Cooking time: 2 hours
Servings: 4

Ingredients:
- 2 tablespoons olive oil
- 2 bunches red chard, roughly chopped
- 3 tablespoons veggie stock
- 2 tablespoons capers
- 1 yellow onion, chopped
- Juice of 1 lemon
- Salt and black pepper to the taste
- 1 teaspoon stevia
- ¼ cup kalamata olives, pitted and chopped

Directions:
Grease your Crockpot with the oil, add red chard, stock, onion, lemon juice, salt, pepper, stevia and olives, toss a bit, cover and cook on High for 2 hours. Add capers, divide between plates and serve as a side dish. Enjoy!

Nutrition: calories 123, fat 4, fiber 3, carbs 4, protein 5

Kale Side Dish

Preparation time: 10 minutes
Cooking time: 2 hours
Servings: 4

Ingredients:
- 1 cup chicken stock
- A pinch of salt and black pepper
- 1 big kale bunch, roughly torn
- 1 tablespoon balsamic vinegar
- 1/3 cup almonds, toasted
- 3 garlic cloves, minced
- 1 small yellow onion, chopped
- 2 tablespoons olive oil

Directions:
Grease your Crockpot with the oil, add kale, stock, vinegar, onion, garlic, salt and pepper, toss, cover and cook on High for 2 hours. Add almonds, toss and serve as a side dish.
Enjoy!

Nutrition: calories 140, fat 6, fiber 3, carbs 5, protein 3

Hungarian Cabbage Side Dish

Preparation time: 10 minutes
Cooking time: 2 hours and 30 minutes
Servings: 4

Ingredients:
- 1 and ½ pound green cabbage, shredded
- Salt and black pepper to the taste
- 3 tablespoons olive oil
- 1 cup veggie stock
- ¼ teaspoon sweet paprika

Directions:
Grease your Crockpot with the oil, add cabbage, salt, pepper, paprika and stock, cover and cook on High for 2 hours and 30 minutes. Divide between plates and serve as a side dish.
Enjoy!

Nutrition: calories 170, fat 4, fiber 2, carbs 5, protein 5

Mushrooms Winter Mix

Preparation time: 10 minutes
Cooking time: 3 hours
Servings: 4

Ingredients:
- 4 tablespoons avocado oil
- 3 tablespoons veggie stock
- 1 teaspoon garlic powder
- 16 ounces baby mushrooms
- Salt and black pepper to the taste
- 3 tablespoons onion, dried
- 3 tablespoons parsley flakes

Directions:
Grease your Crockpot with the oil, add mushrooms, stock, garlic powder, salt, pepper, dried onion and parsley flakes, cover and cook on High for 3 hours. Divide between plates and serve as a side dish.
Enjoy!

Nutrition: calories 192, fat 6, fiber 5, carbs 6, protein 2

Balsamic Swiss Chard with Pine Nuts and Raisins

Preparation time: 10 minutes
Cooking time: 2 hours
Servings: 4

Ingredients:
- 1 bunch Swiss chard, cut into strips
- 2 tablespoons olive oil
- 1 tablespoon balsamic vinegar
- A pinch of salt and black pepper
- ½ small yellow onion, chopped
- ¼ teaspoon red pepper flakes
- ¼ cup pine nuts, toasted
- 2 oz raisins

Directions:
Grease your Crockpot with the oil, add Swiss chard, vinegar, salt, pepper, onion and pepper flakes, cover and cook on High for 2 hours. Add raisins and pine nuts, toss, divide between plates and serve as a side dish. Enjoy!

Nutrition: calories 120, fat 2, fiber 1, carbs 7, protein 4

Balsamic Spinach and Chard

Preparation time: 10 minutes
Cooking time: 2 hours and 20 minutes
Servings: 4

Ingredients:
- 1 yellow onion, sliced
- 4 tablespoons pine nuts, toasted
- 2 tablespoons olive oil
- 6 garlic cloves, chopped
- ¼ cup balsamic vinegar
- 2 and ½ cups baby spinach
- 2 and ½ cups Swiss chard, roughly torn
- Salt and black pepper to the taste
- A pinch of nutmeg

Directions:
Grease your Crockpot with the oil, add onion, garlic, spinach, chard, salt, pepper, nutmeg and vinegar, toss a bit, cover and cook on High for 2 hours and 30 minutes. Add pine nuts, toss, divide between plates and serve as a side dish.
Enjoy!

Nutrition: calories 140, fat 1, fiber 2, carbs 3, protein 3

Cherry Tomatoes Side Dish

Preparation time: 10 minutes
Cooking time: 2 hours
Servings: 6

Ingredients:
- 1 jalapeno pepper, chopped
- 4 garlic cloves, minced
- Salt and black pepper to the taste
- 2 pounds cherry tomatoes, halved
- 1 yellow onion, cut into wedges
- ¼ cup olive oil
- ½ teaspoon oregano, dried
- 1 and ½ cups chicken stock
- ¼ cup basil, chopped
- ½ cup parmesan, grated

Directions:
Grease your Crockpot with the oil, add tomatoes, jalapeno, garlic, salt, pepper, onion, oregano and stock, toss a bit, cover and cook on High for 2 hours. Add parmesan and basil, toss, divide between plates and serve as a side dish.
Enjoy!

Nutrition: calories 120, fat 2, fiber 3, carbs 5, protein 4

Squash Mash

Preparation time: 10 minutes
Cooking time: 4 hours
Servings: 4

Ingredients:
- ½ cup stock
- 2 butternut squash, peeled, roughly cubed and seeds removed
- Salt and black pepper to the taste
- ¼ teaspoon baking soda
- 2 tablespoons avocado oil
- ½ teaspoon nutmeg, ground
- 2 tablespoons stevia

Directions:
In your Crockpot, mix squash with stock, salt, pepper and stevia, cover and cook on Low for 4 hours. Mash squash using a potato masher, add oil, baking soda and nutmeg, whisk well, divide between plates and serve as a side dish.
Enjoy!

Nutrition: calories 152, fat 3, fiber 2, carbs 4, protein 9

Red Chard and Capers

Preparation time: 10 minutes
Cooking time: 3 hours
Servings: 4

Ingredients:
- 2 tablespoons olive oil
- 2 tablespoons chicken stock
- 1 yellow onion, chopped
- 2 tablespoons capers
- Juice of 1 lemon
- Salt and black pepper to the taste
- 1 teaspoon erythritol
- 1 bunch red chard, chopped
- ¼ cup kalamata olives, pitted and chopped

Directions:
Grease your Crockpot with the oil, add chard, stock, onion, salt, pepper, lemon juice and erythritol, toss, cover and cook on Low for 3 hours. Add olives and capers, toss, divide between plates and serve as a side dish.
Enjoy!

Nutrition: calories 119, fat 7, fiber 3, carbs 7, protein 2

Balsamic Kale

Preparation time: 10 minutes
Cooking time: 4 hours
Servings: 4

Ingredients:
- 2 cups veggie stock
- 1 tablespoon balsamic vinegar
- 1/3 cup almonds, toasted
- 3 garlic cloves, minced
- 1 bunch kale, steamed and chopped
- 1 small yellow onion, chopped
- 2 tablespoons olive oil

Directions:
Grease your Crockpot with the oil, add kale, stock, vinegar, garlic and onion, cover and cook on Low for 4 hours. Add almonds, toss, divide between plates and serve as a side dish.
Enjoy!

Nutrition: calories 170, fat 11, fiber 3, carbs 7, protein 7

Simple Broccoli Side Dish

Preparation time: 5 minutes
Cooking time: 4 hours
Servings: 6

Ingredients:
- 31 oz broccoli, florets separated
- 1 cup chicken stock
- 5 lemon slices
- Salt and black pepper to the taste

Directions:
In your Crockpot, mix broccoli with stock, lemon slices, salt and pepper, cover and cook on Low for 4 hours. Divide broccoli between plates and serve as a side dish.
Enjoy!

Nutrition: calories 82, fat 1, fiber 2, carbs 6, protein 3

Fast and Creamy Fennel Mix

Preparation time: 5 minutes
Cooking time: 3 hours
Servings: 3

Ingredients:
- 2 big fennel bulbs, sliced
- 2 tablespoons olive oil
- 1 tablespoon coconut flour
- 2 cups coconut milk
- ¼ teaspoon nutmeg, ground
- Salt and black pepper to the taste.

Directions:
Grease your Crockpot with the oil, add fennel, coconut milk, flour, nutmeg, salt and pepper, toss, cover and cook on High for 3 hours. Divide between plates and serve as a side dish.
Enjoy!

Nutrition: calories 121, fat 2, fiber 3, carbs 6, protein 12

Colored Bell Peppers Mix

Preparation time: 10 minutes
Cooking time: 3 hours
Servings: 4

Ingredients:
- 2 yellow bell peppers, thinly sliced
- 1 green bell pepper, thinly sliced
- 2 red bell peppers, thinly sliced
- 2 tomatoes, chopped
- 2 garlic cloves, minced
- 4 tablespoons chicken stock
- 1 red onion, thinly sliced
- Salt and black pepper to the taste
- 1 bunch parsley, finely chopped
- A drizzle of olive oil

Directions:
Grease your Crockpot with the oil and add yellow, green and red bell peppers. Also add stock, tomatoes, garlic, onion, salt and pepper, cover and cook on High for 3 hours. Add parsley, toss, divide between plates and serve as a side dish.
Enjoy!

Nutrition: calories 152, fat 3, fiber 3, carbs 5, protein 4

Broccoli and Tomatoes Mix

Preparation time: 10 minutes
Cooking time: 4 hours
Servings: 4

Ingredients:
- 1 broccoli head, florets separated
- 2 teaspoons coriander, ground
- A drizzle of olive oil
- 1 yellow onion, chopped
- Salt and black pepper to the taste
- A pinch of red pepper, crushed
- 1 small ginger piece, chopped
- 1 garlic clove, minced
- 28 ounces canned tomatoes, pureed

Directions:
Grease your Crockpot with the oil, add broccoli, coriander, onion, salt, pepper, red pepper, ginger, garlic and tomatoes, toss a bit, cover and cook on Low for 4 hours. Divide between plates and serve as a side dish.
Enjoy!

Nutrition: calories 150, fat 4, fiber 2, carbs 5, protein 12

Bok Choy and Bacon Mix

Preparation time: 10 minutes
Cooking time: 2 hours
Servings: 2

Ingredients:
- 2 garlic cloves, minced
- 2 cup bok choy, chopped
- 4 tablespoons chicken stock
- 2 bacon slices, chopped
- Salt and black pepper to the taste
- A drizzle of avocado oil

Directions:
Grease your Crockpot with the oil, add bok choy, stock, garlic, bacon, salt and pepper, cover and cook on High for 2 hours. Divide between plates and serve as a side dish.
Enjoy!

Nutrition: calories 50, fat 1, fiber 4, carbs 8, protein 8

Creamy Celery Side Dish

Preparation time: 10 minutes
Cooking time: 4 hours
Servings: 8

Ingredients:
- 26 ounces celery leaves and stalks, chopped
- 1 tablespoon onion flakes
- Salt and black pepper to the taste
- 3 teaspoons fenugreek powder
- 3 tablespoons veggie stock
- 6 ounces coconut cream

Directions:
In your Crockpot, mix celery with onion flakes, salt, pepper, fenugreek, stock and cream, cover and cook on Low for 4 hours. Divide between plates and serve as a side dish.
Enjoy!

Nutrition: calories 140, fat 2, fiber 1, carbs 5, protein 10

Stewed Celery Mix

Preparation time: 10 minutes
Cooking time: 4 hours
Servings: 6

Ingredients:
- 1 celery bunch, roughly chopped
- 1 yellow onion, chopped
- 1 bunch green onion, chopped
- 4 garlic cloves, minced
- Salt and black pepper to the taste
- 1 parsley bunch, chopped
- 2 mint bunches, chopped
- 2 cups veggie stock
- 4 tablespoons olive oil

Directions:
Grease your Crockpot with the oil, add celery, onion, green onion, garlic, salt, pepper and stock, cover and cook on Low for 3 hours and 30 minutes. Add parsley and mint, cover and cook on Low for 30 minutes more. Divide between plates and serve as a side dish.
Enjoy!

Nutrition: calories 170, fat 7, fiber 4, carbs 6, protein 10

Lemony Collard Greens

Preparation time: 10 minutes
Cooking time: 3 hours
Servings: 4

Ingredients:
- 2 garlic cloves, minced
- ½ cup veggie stock
- 2 and ½ pounds collard greens, chopped
- 1 teaspoon lemon juice
- 1 tablespoon olive oil
- Salt and black pepper to the taste

Directions:
Grease your Crockpot with the oil, add greens, garlic, stock, lemon juice, salt and pepper, cover and cook on Low for 3 hours. Divide between plates and serve as a side dish.
Enjoy!

Nutrition: calories 151, fat 6, fiber 3, carbs 7, protein 8

Collard Greens, Bacon and Tomatoes

Preparation time: 10 minutes
Cooking time: 3 hours
Servings: 4

Ingredients:
- 1 pound collard greens
- 3 bacon strips, chopped
- ¼ cup cherry tomatoes, halved
- A drizzle of olive oil
- 1 tablespoon balsamic vinegar
- 2 tablespoons chicken stock
- Salt and black pepper to the taste

Directions:
Grease your Crockpot with the oil and add bacon on the bottom. Add collard greens, tomatoes, vinegar, stock, salt and pepper, cover and cook on Low for 3 hours. Divide between plates and serve as a side dish. Enjoy!

Nutrition: calories 120, fat 8, fiber 1, carbs 3, protein 7

Mustard Greens and Garlic

Preparation time: 5 minutes
Cooking time: 2 hours
Servings: 4

Ingredients:
- 2 garlic cloves, minced
- 1 pound mustard greens, roughly torn
- 1 tablespoon olive oil
- ½ cup yellow onion, sliced
- Salt and black pepper to the taste
- ¼ cup veggie stock
- ¼ teaspoon avocado oil

Directions:
Grease Crockpot with the olive oil, add garlic, greens, onion, salt, pepper and stock, cover and cook on High for 2 hours. Add avocado oil, toss, divide between plates and serve as a side dish. Enjoy!

Nutrition: calories 120, fat 3, fiber 1, carbs 3, protein 6

Cheesy Collard Greens

Preparation time: 10 minutes
Cooking time: 2 hours and 40 minutes
Servings: 6

Ingredients:
- 1 tablespoon jalapeno pepper, chopped
- 6 eggs, whisked
- 3 tablespoons olive oil
- 1 yellow onion, chopped
- 2 garlic cloves, minced
- 6 bacon slices, chopped
- 3 bunches collard greens, chopped
- ½ cup chicken stock
- Salt and black pepper to the taste
- 1 tablespoon lime juice
- 1 tablespoon cheddar cheese

Directions:
Add the oil to your Crockpot and arrange jalapeno on the bottom. Add onion, garlic, bacon, collard greens, stock, salt, pepper, lime juice and whisked eggs, toss, cover and cook on High for 2 hours and 40 minutes. Add cheese, toss until it melts, divide between plates and serve as a side dish.
Enjoy!

Nutrition: calories 245, fat 13, fiber 1, carbs 5, protein 12

Spring Green Mix

Preparation time: 10 minutes
Cooking time: 4 hours
Servings: 4

Ingredients:
- 2 cups mustard greens, chopped
- 2 cups collard greens, chopped
- 2 cups veggie stock
- 1 yellow onion, chopped
- Salt and black pepper to the taste
- 2 tablespoons coconut aminos
- 2 teaspoons ginger, grated

Directions:
In your Crockpot, mix mustard greens with collard greens, stock, onion, salt, pepper, aminos and ginger, toss, cover and cook on Low for 4 hours. Divide between plates and serve as a side dish.
Enjoy!

Nutrition: calories 140, fat 2, fiber 1, carbs 3, protein 12

Easy Asparagus

Preparation time: 10 minutes
Cooking time: 2 hours and 30 minutes
Servings: 3

Ingredients:
- 10 ounces asparagus spears, cut into medium pieces and steamed
- Salt and black pepper to the taste
- 2 tablespoons parmesan, grated
- 1/3 cup Monterey jack cheese, shredded
- 2 tablespoons mustard
- 4 ounces coconut cream
- 3 tablespoons bacon, cooked and crumbled

Directions:
In your Crockpot, mix asparagus with salt, pepper, mustard, cream and bacon, cover and cook on High for 2 hours and 30 minutes. Add Monterey jack and parmesan cheese, toss until cheese melts, divide between plates and serve as a side dish.
Enjoy!

Nutrition: calories 206, fat 13, fiber 2, carbs 5, protein 13

Spanish Spinach Mix

Preparation time: 10 minutes
Cooking time: 3 hours
Servings: 4

Ingredients:
- 1 yellow onion, sliced
- 3 tablespoons avocado oil
- ¼ cup chicken stock
- 6 garlic cloves, chopped
- ¼ cup pine nuts, toasted
- ¼ cup balsamic vinegar
- ½ teaspoon nutmeg, ground
- 5 cups mixed spinach and chard
- Salt and black pepper to the taste

Directions:
Grease your Crockpot with the oil, add onion, stock, garlic, vinegar, nutmeg, spinach, salt and pepper, toss a bit, cover and cook on High for 3 hours. Add pine nuts, toss, divide between plates and serve as a side dish.
Enjoy!

Nutrition: calories 120, fat 1, fiber 2, carbs 3, protein 6

Squash and Swiss Chard Mix

Preparation time: 10 minutes
Cooking time: 2 hours
Servings: 4

Ingredients:
- 1 red onion, chopped
- 1 bunch Swiss chard, roughly chopped
- 1 butternut squash, cubed
- 1 zucchini, cubed
- 1 green bell pepper, chopped
- Salt and black pepper to the taste
- 4 cups tomatoes, chopped
- 1 cup cauliflower florets, chopped
- 2 cups chicken stock
- 3 ounces fresh tomato puree
- 1 pound turkey fillet, chopped
- 2 garlic cloves, minced
- 2 teaspoons thyme, chopped
- 1 teaspoon rosemary, dried
- 1 tablespoon fennel, minced
- ½ teaspoon red pepper flake

Directions:
Heat up a pan over medium- high heat, add turkey fillet and garlic, stir and cook until it browns and transfer along with its juices to your Crockpot. Add onion, Swiss chard, squash, bell pepper, zucchini, tomatoes, cauliflower, fresh tomato puree, stock, thyme, fennel, rosemary, pepper flakes, salt and pepper, stir, cover and cook on High for 2 hours. Divide between plates and serve as a side dish.
Enjoy!

Nutrition: calories 190, fat 8, fiber 2, carbs 4, protein 9

Simple Cherry Tomatoes and Onion Mix

Preparation time: 10 minutes
Cooking time: 4 hours
Servings: 5

Ingredients:
- 4 garlic cloves, minced
- 2 pounds cherry tomatoes, halved
- ½ red onion, cut into wedges
- Salt and black pepper to the taste
- 3 tablespoons avocado oil
- ½ teaspoon basil, dried
- 1 and ½ cups veggie stock
- ¼ cup parsley, chopped
- ½ cup goat cheese, crumbled

Directions:
Grease your Crockpot with the oil, add garlic, tomatoes, onion wedges, salt, pepper, basil and stock, cover and cook on Low for 4 hours. Divide between plates and serve as a side dish with parsley and goat cheese crumbled on top.
Enjoy!

Nutrition: calories 140, fat 2, fiber 2, carbs 5, protein 8

Creamy Eggplant and Tomatoes

Preparation time: 10 minutes
Cooking time: 5 hours
Servings: 4

Ingredients:

- 4 tomatoes, cut into wedges
- 1 teaspoon garlic, minced
- ¼ yellow onion, chopped
- Salt and black pepper to the taste
- 1 cup chicken stock
- 1 bay leaf
- ½ cup coconut cream
- 2 tablespoons basil, chopped
- 4 tablespoons parmesan, grated
- 1 tablespoon olive oil
- 1 eggplant, cut into medium pieces

Directions:
Grease your Crockpot with the oil, add tomatoes, garlic, onion, salt, pepper, stock, bay leaf, coconut cream, basil and eggplant, cover and cook on Low for 5 hours. Add parmesan, toss, divide between plates and serve as a side dish.
Enjoy!

Nutrition: calories 180, fat 2, fiber 3, carbs 5, protein 10

Creamy Radish Mix

Preparation time: 10 minutes
Cooking time: 3 hours
Servings: 2

Ingredients:

- 14 ounces radishes, halved
- 4 tablespoons coconut cream
- 4 bacon slices, chopped
- 1 tablespoon green onion, chopped
- 1 tablespoon cheddar cheese, grated
- Salt and black pepper to the taste

Directions:
In your Crockpot, mix radishes with cream, bacon, green onion, salt and pepper, toss, cover and cook on High for 3 hours. Divide between plates and serve as a side dish with cheese sprinkled on top.
Enjoy!

Nutrition: calories 340, fat 23, fiber 3, carbs 6, protein 15

Snack and Appetizer Recipes

Simple Cashew Spread

Preparation time: 10 minutes
Cooking time: 6 hours
Servings: 4

Ingredients:
- 5 tablespoons cashews, soaked for 12 hours and blended
- 1 teaspoon apple cider vinegar
- 1 cup veggie stock
- 1 tablespoon water

Directions:
In your Crockpot, mix cashews and stock, stir, cover and cook on Low for 6 hours. Drain, transfer to your food processor, add vinegar and water, pulse well, divide between bowls and serve as a party spread. Enjoy!

Nutrition: calories 221, fat 6, fiber 5, carbs 9, protein 3

Beef Party Rolls

Preparation time: 10 minutes
Cooking time: 8 hours
Servings: 4

Ingredients:
- ½ pounds beef, minced
- 1 green cabbage head, leaves separated
- ½ cup onion, chopped
- 1 cup cauliflower rice
- 2 ounces white mushrooms, chopped
- ¼ cup pine nuts, toasted
- 2 garlic cloves, minced
- 2 tablespoons dill, chopped
- 1 tablespoon olive oil
- 25 ounces tomato sauce
- A pinch of salt and black pepper
- ¼ cup water

Directions:
In a bowl, mix beef with onion, cauliflower, mushrooms, pine nuts, garlic, dill, salt and pepper and stir. Arrange cabbage leaves on a working surface, divide beef mix and wrap them well. Add sauce and water to your Crockpot, stir, add cabbage rolls, cover and cook on Low for 8 hours. Arrange rolls on a platter and serve as an appetizer with some of the sauce from the pot drizzled all over. Enjoy!

Nutrition: calories 361, fat 6, fiber 6, carbs 12, protein 3

Eggplant and Tomato Salsa

Preparation time: 10 minutes
Cooking time: 7 hours
Servings: 4

Ingredients:
- 1 and ½ cups tomatoes, chopped
- 3 cups eggplant, cubed
- 2 teaspoons capers
- 6 ounces green olives, pitted and sliced
- 4 garlic cloves, minced
- 2 teaspoons balsamic vinegar
- 1 tablespoon basil, chopped
- Salt and black pepper to the taste

Directions:
In your Crockpot, mix tomatoes with eggplant, capers, green olives, garlic, vinegar, basil, salt and pepper, toss, cover and cook on Low for 7 hours. Divide salsa Into small bowls and serve as an appetizer.
Enjoy!

Nutrition: calories 200, fat 6, fiber 5, carbs 9, protein 2

Squash and Cauliflower Spread

Preparation time: 10 minutes
Cooking time: 7 hours
Servings: 4

Ingredients:
- 1 cup butternut squash, sliced
- 1 and ½ cups cauliflower florets
- 1/3 cup cashews, soaked for a couple of hours and drained
- ½ cup turnips, chopped
- 2 and ½ cups water
- 1 cup coconut milk
- 1 teaspoon garlic powder
- ¼ cup nutritional yeast
- ¼ teaspoon smoked paprika
- ¼ teaspoon mustard powder
- A pinch of salt and black pepper

Directions:
In your Crockpot, mix squash with cauliflower, cashews, turnips and water, stir, cover and cook on Low for 7 hours. Drain, transfer to a blender, add milk, garlic powder, yeast, paprika, mustard powder, salt and pepper, blend well, divide between bowls and serve as a party spread.
Enjoy!

Nutrition: calories 291, fat 7, fiber 4, carbs 14, protein 3

Mixed Veggies Spread

Preparation time: 10 minutes
Cooking time: 5 hours
Servings: 7

Ingredients:
- ½ cauliflower head, riced
- 34 ounces canned tomatoes, crushed
- 10 ounces white mushrooms, chopped
- 1 cup butternut squash, shredded
- 2 cups eggplant, cubed
- 6 garlic cloves, minced
- 2 tablespoons sugar-free maple syrup
- 2 tablespoons balsamic vinegar
- 2 tablespoons fresh tomato puree
- 1 tablespoon basil, chopped
- 1 and ½ tablespoons oregano, chopped
- 1 and ½ teaspoons rosemary, dried
- A pinch of salt and black pepper

Directions:
In your Crockpot, mix cauliflower with tomatoes, mushrooms, squash, eggplant, garlic, maple syrup, vinegar, fresh tomato puree, rosemary, salt and pepper, stir, cover and cook on High for 5 hours. Add basil and oregano, stir again, blend a bit using an immersion blender, divide between bowls and serve as a spread.
Enjoy!

Nutrition: calories 301, fat 7, fiber 6, carbs 10, protein 6

Cashew Hummus

Preparation time: 10 minutes
Cooking time: 3 hours
Servings: 4

Ingredients:
- 1 cup water
- 1 cup cashews
- 2 tablespoons tahini paste
- ¼ teaspoon garlic powder
- ¼ teaspoon onion powder
- ¼ cup nutritional yeast
- A pinch of salt and black pepper
- ¼ teaspoon mustard powder
- 1 teaspoon apple cider vinegar

Directions:
In your Crockpot, mix water with cashews, yeast, salt and pepper, stir, cover and cook on High for 3 hours. Transfer to your blender, add tahini, garlic powder, onion powder, mustard powder and vinegar, pulse well, divide between bowls and serve.
Enjoy!

Nutrition: calories 192, fat 7, fiber 7, carbs 12, protein 4

Spinach and Chestnuts Dip

Preparation time: 10 minutes
Cooking time: 1 hour
Servings: 4

Ingredients:
- 1 cup coconut cream
- 10 ounces spinach, torn
- 8 ounces water chestnuts, chopped
- 1 garlic clove, minced
- Black pepper to the taste

Directions:
In your Crockpot, mix coconut cream with spinach, chestnuts, black pepper and garlic, stir, cover and cook on High for 30 minutes. Blend using an immersion blender, divide between bowls and serve as a party dip. Enjoy!

Nutrition: calories 241, fat 5, fiber 7, carbs 12, protein 5

Bell Peppers Appetizer

Preparation time: 10 minutes
Cooking time: 4 hours and 10 minutes
Servings: 5

Ingredients:
- ½ yellow onion, chopped
- 2 teaspoons olive oil
- 2 celery ribs, chopped
- 1 tablespoon chili powder
- 3 garlic cloves, minced
- 2 teaspoon cumin, ground
- 1 and ½ teaspoon oregano, dried
- 2 and ½ cups cauliflower rice
- 1 tomato chopped
- 1 chipotle pepper
- A pinch of salt and black pepper
- 5 colored bell peppers, tops and Insides scooped out
- ½ cup tomato sauce

Directions:
Heat up a pan with the oil over medium- high heat, add onion and celery, stir and cook for 5 minutes. Add garlic, chili, cumin, oregano, cauliflower, tomato, chipotle, salt and pepper, stir, cook for a couple of minutes more, take off heat and stuff peppers with this mix. Arrange bell peppers in your Crockpot, spread tomato sauce over them, cover, cook on Low for 4 hours, arrange on a platter and serve them as an appetizer. Enjoy!

Nutrition: calories 221, fat 5, fiber 4, carbs 9, protein 3

Artichoke and Coconut Spread

Preparation time: 10 minutes
Cooking time: 2 hours
Servings: 8

Ingredients:

- 28 ounces canned artichokes, drained and chopped
- 10 ounces spinach
- 8 ounces coconut cream
- 1 yellow onion, chopped
- 2 garlic cloves, minced
- ¾ cup coconut milk
- ½ cup feta cheese, crumbled
- 1/3 cup mayonnaise
- 1 tablespoon red vinegar
- A pinch of salt and black pepper

Directions:
In your Crockpot, mix artichokes with spinach, coconut cream, onion, garlic, coconut milk, cheese, mayo, vinegar, salt and pepper, stir well, cover and cook on Low for 2 hours. Whisk spread well, divide between bowls and serve as an appetizer.
Enjoy!

Nutrition: calories 305, fat 14, fiber 4, carbs 9, protein 13

Mushroom and Bell Peppers Spread

Preparation time: 10 minutes
Cooking time: 4 hours
Servings: 6

Ingredients:

- 2 cups green bell peppers, chopped
- 1 cup yellow onion, chopped
- 3 garlic cloves, minced
- 1 pound mushrooms, chopped
- 28 ounces tomato sauce
- Salt and black pepper to the taste

Directions:
In your Crockpot, mix bell peppers with onion, garlic, mushrooms, tomato sauce, salt and pepper, stir, cover and cook on Low for 4 hours. Divide between bowls and serve as a spread.
Enjoy!

Nutrition: calories 205, fat 4, fiber 7, carbs 9, protein 3

Chicken Wings Appetizer

Preparation time: 10 minutes
Cooking time: 3 hours
Servings: 6

Ingredients:
- 2 tablespoons garlic, minced
- 2 cups water
- 3 tablespoons coconut aminos
- 1 tablespoon ginger, minced
- 1 teaspoon olive oil
- A pinch of salt and black pepper
- 3 pounds chicken wings
- A pinch of red pepper flakes, crushed
- 2 tablespoons five spice powder
- Chopped cilantro, for serving

Directions:
Put water in your Crockpot, add oil, salt, pepper, aminos, ginger and garlic and whisk well. Add chicken wings, pepper flakes and five spice, toss, cover and cook on High for 3 hours. Arrange chicken wings on a platter, drizzle some of the sauce over them, sprinkle cilantro and serve as an appetizer.
Enjoy!

Nutrition: calories 252, fat 4, fiber 4, carbs 9, protein 20

Cod Sticks

Preparation time: 10 minutes
Cooking time: 2 hours
Servings: 4

Ingredients:
- 2 eggs, whisked
- 1 pound cod fillets, cut into medium strips
- 1 and ½ cups almond flour
- A pinch of salt and black pepper to the taste
- ½ cup tapioca flour
- ¼ teaspoon paprika
- Cooking spray

Directions:
In a bowl, mix almond flour, salt, pepper, tapioca and paprika and stir. Put the eggs In another bowl. Dip fish sticks In the egg, dredge In flour mix, arrange them In your Crockpot after you've greased it with cooking spray, cover and cook on High for 2 hours. Arrange cod sticks on a platter and serve.
Enjoy!

Nutrition: calories 261, fat 2, fiber 4, carbs 7, protein 12

Pecans Snack

Preparation time: 10 minutes
Cooking time: 2 hours and 20 minutes
Servings: 10

Ingredients:
- 1 pound pecans, halved
- 2 tablespoons olive oil
- 1 teaspoon basil, dried
- 1 tablespoon chili powder
- 1 teaspoon oregano, dried
- ¼ teaspoon garlic powder
- 1 teaspoon thyme, dried
- ½ teaspoon onion powder

Directions:
In your Crockpot, mix pecans with oil, basil, chili powder, oregano, garlic powder, onion powder and thyme, toss to coat, cover, cook on High for 20 minutes and on Low for 2 hours. Divide between bowls and serve as a snack.
Enjoy!

Nutrition: calories 78, fat 3, fiber 2, carbs 9, protein 2

Party Meatballs

Preparation time: 10 minutes
Cooking time: 4 hours
Servings: 4

Ingredients:
- 1 and ½ pounds beef, ground
- 2 small yellow onions, chopped
- 1 egg
- A pinch of salt and black pepper
- 3 tablespoons cilantro, chopped
- 14 ounces canned coconut milk
- 2 tablespoons tomato passata
- 1 teaspoon basil, dried
- 1 tablespoon green curry paste
- 1 tablespoon coconut aminos

Directions:
Put the meat In a bowl, add onions, egg, salt, pepper and 1 tablespoon cilantro, stir well, shape medium sized meatballs and place them In your Crockpot. Add tomato passata, aminos, coconut milk, curry paste, the rest of the cilantro and basil, toss to cover all meatballs and cook on Low for 4 hours. Arrange meatballs on a platter and serve them as an appetizer.
Enjoy!

Nutrition: calories 260, fat 6, fiber 2, carbs 8, protein 4

Shrimp, Mussels and Clams Appetizer

Preparation time: 10 minutes
Cooking time: 6 hours
Servings: 4

Ingredients:
- 1 pound shrimp, peeled and deveined
- 2 pounds mussels, cleaned and debearded
- 28 ounces canned clams
- 1 yellow onion, chopped
- 10 ounces fresh tomato puree

Directions:
In your Crockpot, mix shrimp with mussels, clams, onion and fresh tomato puree, stir, cover and cook on Low for 6 hours. Divide Into small bowls and serve as an appetizer.
Enjoy!

Nutrition: calories 200, fat 3, fiber 2, carbs 7, protein 5

Curried Shrimp Appetizer

Preparation time: 10 minutes
Cooking time: 4 hours and 30 minutes
Servings: 2

Ingredients:
- ½ small yellow onion, chopped
- 1 pound shrimp, deveined and peeled
- 2 garlic cloves, minced
- 1 small green bell pepper, chopped
- 8 ounces canned coconut milk
- 3 tablespoons fresh tomato puree
- ½ teaspoon red pepper, crushed
- ¾ tablespoons curry powder

Directions:
In your food processor, mix onion with garlic, bell pepper, fresh tomato puree, coconut milk, red pepper and curry powder, blend well, add to your Crockpot, cover and cook on Low for 4 hours. Add shrimp, stir and cook on Low for 30 minutes more. Divide between bowls and serve as an appetizer.
Enjoy!

Nutrition: calories 200, fat 4, fiber 3, carbs 4, protein 5

Stuffed Chicken Breast Appetizer

Preparation time: 10 minutes
Cooking time: 6 hours
Servings: 4

Ingredients:
- 4 chicken breasts, skinless and boneless
- 1 tablespoon olive oil
- 1 small yellow onion, chopped
- 2 chili peppers, chopped
- 1 small red bell pepper, chopped
- 2 teaspoons garlic, minced
- 6 ounces spinach
- 1 and ½ teaspoon oregano, chopped
- 1 tablespoon lemon juice
- 1 cup veggie stock
- A pinch of salt and black pepper
- A handful parsley, chopped

Directions:
Heat up a pan with the oil over medium- high heat, add bell pepper, chili peppers and onions, stir and cook for 3 minutes. Add spinach, garlic, salt, pepper and oregano, stir, cook for a couple more seconds and take off heat. Cut a pocket In each chicken breast, stuff with spinach mix, arrange In your Crockpot, add stock over them, cover and cook on Low for 6 hours. Arrange stuffed chicken on a platter, sprinkle parsley on top, drizzle the lemon juice and serve.
Enjoy!

Nutrition: calories 245, fat 4, fiber 3, carbs 8, protein 14

Pecans Snack

Preparation time: 10 minutes
Cooking time: 3 hours
Servings: 8

Ingredients:
- 1 cup stevia
- 1 and ½ tablespoon cinnamon powder
- 1 egg white
- 2 teaspoons vanilla extract
- 4 cups pecans
- ¼ cup water
- Cooking spray

Directions:
In a bowl, mix stevia with cinnamon and stir. In another bowl, mix the egg white with vanilla and whisk well. Grease your Crockpot with cooking spray, add pecans, egg white mix and stevia mix as well, toss, cover and cook on Low for 3 hours. Divide pecans mix Into bowls and serve as a snack.
Enjoy!

Nutrition: calories 172, fat 3, fiber 5, carbs 8, protein 2

Spicy Cauliflower Dip

Preparation time: 10 minutes
Cooking time: 2 hours and 15 minutes
Servings: 6

Ingredients:
- 4 bacon slices, chopped and cooked
- 2 jalapenos, chopped
- ½ cup coconut cream
- 2 cups cauliflower rice
- ¼ cup cheddar cheese, grated
- A pinch of salt and black pepper
- 2 tablespoons chives, chopped

Directions:
In your Crockpot, mix bacon with jalapenos, coconut cream, cauliflower, salt and pepper, stir, cover and cook on Low for 2 hours. Add cashew cheese and chives, cover, cook on Low for 15 minutes more, divide between bowls and serve as a party dip
Enjoy!

Nutrition: calories 242, fat 3, fiber 3, carbs 7, protein 6

Spicy Nuts Mix

Preparation time: 10 minutes
Cooking time: 4 hours
Servings: 20

Ingredients:
- 4 tablespoons coconut oil, melted
- 1 ounce Italian seasoning
- 1 teaspoon cinnamon powder
- Cayenne pepper to the taste
- 2 cups cashews
- 2 cups pecans
- 2 cups almonds
- 2 cups walnuts

Directions:
In your Crockpot, mix oil with Italian seasoning, cinnamon, cayenne, cashews, pecans, almonds and walnuts, toss well, cover, cook on Low for 4 hours, divide between bowls and serve as a party snack.
Enjoy!

Nutrition: calories 200, fat 4, fiber 3, carbs 7, protein 4

Veggie Party Mix

Preparation time: 10 minutes
Cooking time: 2 hours
Servings: 8

Ingredients:
- 2 eggplants, cubed
- 3 celery stalks, chopped
- 1 pound plum tomatoes, chopped
- 1 zucchini, halved and sliced
- 1 red bell pepper, chopped
- 1/3 cup sweet onion, chopped
- 3 tablespoons fresh tomato puree
- 1 tablespoon stevia
- 1 teaspoon red pepper flakes, crushed
- ¼ cup basil, chopped
- ¼ cup parsley, chopped
- A pinch of salt and black pepper
- ¼ cup green olives, pitted and chopped
- ¼ cup capers
- 2 tablespoons red wine vinegar

Directions:
In your Crockpot, mix the eggplants with celery, tomatoes, zucchini, bell pepper, sweet onion, fresh tomato puree, stevia, pepper flakes, basil, parsley, salt, pepper, olives, capers and vinegar, stir, cover, cook on High for 2 hours, divide between bowls and serve as an appetizer.
Enjoy!

Nutrition: calories 80, fat 1, fiber 2, carbs 6, protein 1

Walnuts and Pumpkin Seeds Snack

Preparation time: 10 minutes
Cooking time: 2 hours and 30 minutes
Servings: 12

Ingredients:
- Cooking spray
- 1 cup walnuts, chopped
- 1 cup pumpkin seeds
- 2 tablespoons dill, dried
- 2 tablespoons olive oil
- 1 teaspoon rosemary, dried
- 1 tablespoon lemon peel, grated

Directions:
Grease your Crockpot with cooking spray, add walnuts, pumpkin seeds, oil, dill, rosemary and lemon peel, toss, cover and cook on Low for 2 hours and 30 minutes. Divide into bowls and serve as a snack.
Enjoy!

Nutrition: calories 100, fat 2, fiber 2, carbs 3, protein 2

Coconut Crab Spread

Preparation time: 10 minutes
Cooking time: 2 hours
Servings: 6

Ingredients:
- 4 ounces coconut cream
- 1 pound crab meat
- 1 jalapeno, chopped
- 1 red bell pepper, chopped
- 4 tablespoons lemon juice
- 2 garlic cloves, minced
- ½ teaspoon mustard powder

Directions:
In your Crockpot, mix cream with crab meat, jalapeno, bell pepper, lemon juice, garlic and mustard, stir, cover and cook on High for 2 hours. Blend using your immersion blender, divide between bowls and serve as a spread.
Enjoy!

Nutrition: calories 202, fat 3, fiber 6, carbs 7, protein 3

Tomato and Sweet Onion Dip

Preparation time: 10 minutes
Cooking time: 5 hours
Servings: 12

Ingredients:
- 8 pounds tomatoes, peeled and chopped
- 1 sweet onion, chopped
- 6 garlic cloves, minced
- 6 ounces fresh tomato puree
- ¼ cup white vinegar
- 2 tablespoons stevia
- 1 and ½ tablespoons Italian seasoning
- A pinch of salt and black pepper
- ½ cup basil, chopped
- 1 tablespoon thyme, chopped

Directions:
In your Crockpot, mix tomatoes with onions, garlic, fresh tomato puree, vinegar, stevia, Italian seasoning, salt, pepper, basil and thyme, stir, cover, cook on High for 5 hours, blend using an immersion blender, divide between bowls and serve as a dip.
Enjoy!

Nutrition: calories 182, fat 3, fiber 6, carbs 8, protein 3

Mussels and Veggies Appetizer

Preparation time: 10 minutes
Cooking time: 2 hours
Servings: 4

Ingredients:
- 2 pounds mussels, scrubbed
- 2 tablespoons olive oil
- 1 yellow onion, chopped
- 1 teaspoon parsley, dried
- 1 zucchini, sliced
- ½ teaspoon red pepper flakes, crushed
- 2 teaspoons garlic, minced
- 14 ounces tomatoes, chopped
- ½ cup chicken stock

Directions:
In your Crockpot, mix mussels with oil, onion parsley, pepper flakes, garlic, zucchini, tomatoes and stock, stir, cover and cook on High for 2 hours. Divide between bowls and serve as an appetizer.
Enjoy!

Nutrition: calories 230, fat 2, fiber 3, carbs 7, protein 2

Cheese Dip

Preparation time: 10 minutes
Cooking time: 2 hours and 30 minutes
Servings: 13

Ingredients:
- 8 ounces cream cheese
- A pinch of salt and black pepper
- 16 ounces coconut cream
- 8 ounces pepper jack cheese, chopped
- 15 ounces canned tomatoes mixed with habaneros
- 1 pound boiled turkey fillet, ground
- ¼ cup green onions, chopped

Directions:
Heat up a pan over medium heat, add turkey, stir, brown for a few minutes and transfer to your Crockpot. Add tomatoes mixed with habaneros, salt, pepper, green onions, pepper jack cheese, cream cheese and coconut cream, cover and cook on High for 2 hours and 30 minutes. Stir your dip really well, divide between bowls and serve.
Enjoy!

Nutrition: calories 184, fat 12, fiber 1, carbs 3, protein 6

Different Cream Cheese Dip

Preparation time: 10 minutes
Cooking time: 2 hours
Servings: 4

Ingredients:
- 4 ounces cream cheese, soft
- ½ cup mozzarella cheese, shredded
- ¼ cup parmesan, grated
- ¼ cup coconut cream
- Salt and black pepper to the taste
- 1/2 cup tomato sauce
- ¼ cup mayonnaise
- 1 tablespoon green bell pepper, chopped
- 6 pepperoni slices, chopped
- 4 black olives, pitted and chopped

Directions:
In your Crockpot, mix cream cheese with mozzarella, parmesan, cream, salt, pepper, tomato sauce, mayo, bell pepper, Italian seasoning and pepperoni, cover and cook on High for 2 hours. Divide dip Into bowls, sprinkle olives all over and serve.
Enjoy!

Nutrition: calories 400, fat 14, fiber 4, carbs 4, protein 15

Zucchini and Tomato Dip

Preparation time: 10 minutes
Cooking time: 2 hours
Servings: 4

Ingredients:
- 1 cup mozzarella, shredded
- ¼ cup tomato sauce
- 3 zucchinis, roughly chopped
- Salt and black pepper to the taste
- A pinch of cumin
- Cooking spray

Directions:
Spray your Crockpot with cooking spray, add zucchinis, tomato sauce, salt, pepper and cumin, cover and cook on High for 2 hours. Add mozzarella, stir really well, blend a bit using your immersion blender, divide Into small bowls and serve as a dip.
Enjoy!

Nutrition: calories 140, fat 4, fiber 2, carbs 6, protein 4

Zucchini Hummus

Preparation time: 10 minutes
Cooking time: 2 hours
Servings: 5

Ingredients:
- 4 cups zucchinis, chopped
- 1 cup chicken stock
- ¼ cup olive oil
- Salt and black pepper to the taste
- 4 garlic cloves, minced
- ¾ cup tahini
- ½ cup lemon juice
- 1 tablespoon cumin, ground

Directions:
In your Crockpot, mix zucchinis with stock, salt, pepper and cumin, cover, cook on High for 2 hours and transfer to your blender, Add oil, garlic, lemon juice and tahini, blend really well, divide Into small bowls and serve.
Enjoy!

Nutrition: calories 80, fat 5, fiber 3, carbs 6, protein 7

Beef Jerky Snack

Preparation time: 6 hours
Cooking time: 5 hours
Servings: 6

Ingredients:
- 2 cups chicken stock
- ½ cup soy sauce
- 2 tablespoons black peppercorns
- 2 tablespoons black pepper
- 2 pounds beef round, sliced

Directions:
In a bowl, mix soy sauce with black peppercorns, black pepper and whisk well. Add beef slices, toss to coat, leave aside in the fridge for 6 hours, transfer everything to your Crockpot, pour with chicken stock, cover and cook on Low for 5 hours. Divide between bowls and serve.
Enjoy!

Nutrition: calories 300, fat 12, fiber 4, carbs 10, protein 8

Stuffed Mushrooms

Preparation time: 10 minutes
Cooking time: 4 hours
Servings: 5

Ingredients:
- ¼ cup mayonnaise
- 1 teaspoon garlic powder
- 1 cup chicken stock
- 1 small yellow onion, chopped
- 14 ounces white mushroom caps
- Salt and black pepper to the taste
- 1 teaspoon curry powder
- 4 ounces cream cheese, soft
- ¼ cup coconut cream
- ½ cup Mexican cheese, shredded
- 1 cup shrimp, cooked, peeled, deveined and chopped

Directions:
In a bowl, mix mayo with garlic powder, onion, curry powder, cream cheese, coconut cream, cheese, shrimp, salt and pepper to the taste, whisk well and stuff mushrooms with this mix. Transfer mushrooms to your Crockpot, add the stock over them, cover and cook on Low for 4 hours. Arrange mushrooms on a platter and serve as an appetizer.
Enjoy!

Nutrition: calories 244, fat 20, fiber 3, carbs 7, protein 14

Cheesy Party Wings

Preparation time: 10 minutes
Cooking time: 5 hours
Servings: 6

Ingredients:
- 6 pounds chicken wings, halved
- 3 tablespoons chicken stock
- Salt and black pepper to the taste
- ½ teaspoon Italian seasoning
- 2 tablespoons olive oil
- ½ cup parmesan cheese, grated
- A pinch of red pepper flakes, crushed
- 1 teaspoon garlic powder

Directions:
Grease your Crockpot with the oil, add chicken wings, salt, pepper, Italian seasoning, pepper flakes, garlic powder and stock, cover and cook on Low for 5 hours. Add parmesan, toss, divide chicken wings between plates and serve as an appetizer.
Enjoy!

Nutrition: calories 134, fat 8, fiber 1, carbs 5, protein 14

Chicken Rolls

Preparation time: 2 hours
Cooking time: 2 hours and 30 minutes
Servings: 12

Ingredients:
- 4 ounces blue cheese, crumbled
- 2 cups chicken, cooked and finely chopped
- Salt and black pepper to the taste
- 2 green onions, chopped
- 2 celery stalks, finely chopped
- 1 cup tomato sauce
- ½ teaspoon erythritol
- 2 tablespoons olive oil

For egg roll wrappers:
- 3 eggs, beaten 3/4 cup cold water
- 1 teaspoon salt
- 4 cups coconut flour
- 5 tablespoons olive oil

Directions:
For wrappers, mix all the ingredients. Heat a wok over medium-high heat, thinly coat with olive oil, pour 1/12 of the egg mixture in approximately 7 inch circle. Cook 1 minute, remove from heat, repeat with remaining mixture. In a bowl, mix chicken meat with blue cheese, salt, pepper, green onions, celery, tomato sauce, and sweetener, stir well, and keep in the refrigerator for 2 hours. Place egg wrappers on a working surface, divide chicken mixture on them, roll, and seal edges. Heat a pan with vegetable oil over medium-high heat, add egg rolls, cook until they are golden, flip, and cook on the other side as well. Arrange on a platter and serve them.
Enjoy!

Nutrition: calories 220, fat 7, fiber 2, carbs 6, protein 10

Zucchini and Cheese Rolls

Preparation time: 10 minutes
Cooking time: 1 hour
Servings: 24

Ingredients:
- 2 tablespoons olive oil
- 3 zucchinis, thinly sliced
- ½ cup tomato sauce
- 24 basil leaves
- 2 tablespoons mint, chopped
- 1 and 1/3 cup ricotta cheese
- Salt and black pepper to the taste
- ¼ cup basil leaves, whole

Directions:
Brush zucchini slices with half of the olive oil, season with salt and pepper, place them on a working surface and leave aside for now. In a bowl, mix ricotta with chopped basil, mint, salt and pepper and stir well. Spread this over zucchini slices, divide whole basil leaves as well, roll, transfer to your Crockpot, add the rest of the oil and the tomato sauce over them, cover and cook on High for 1 hour. Arrange on a platter and serve as an appetizer.
Enjoy!

Nutrition: calories 100, fat 3, fiber 3, carbs 6, protein 2

Salmon Cakes

Preparation time: 10 minutes
Cooking time: 2 hours
Servings: 4

Ingredients:
- 2 garlic cloves, minced
- 1 yellow onion, chopped
- 1 pound wild salmon, boneless and minced
- ¼ cup chives, chopped
- 1 egg
- 2 tablespoons Dijon mustard
- 1 tablespoon coconut flour
- Salt and black pepper to the taste

For the sauce:
- 4 garlic cloves, minced
- 2 tablespoons olive oil
- 2 tablespoons Dijon mustard
- Juice and zest of 1 lemon
- 2 cups coconut cream
- 2 tablespoons chives, chopped

Directions:
In a bowl, mix onion, 2 garlic cloves, salmon, ¼ cup chives, coconut flour, salt, pepper, 2 tablespoons mustard and egg and stir well. Shape medium cakes and put them In your Crockpot. Add 4 garlic cloves, the oil, 2 tablespoons mustard, lemon zest, lemon juice, coconut cream and chives, cover and cook on High for 2 hours. Arrange salmon meatballs on a platter, drizzle some of the cooking sauce over them and serve as an appetizer.
Enjoy!

Nutrition: calories 171, fat 5, fiber 1, carbs 6, protein 16

Salmon Salsa

Preparation time: 30 minutes
Cooking time: 1 hour
Servings: 4

Ingredients:
- 4 salmon fillets, skinless, boneless and cubed
- 1 tablespoon olive oil
- A pinch of salt and black pepper
- 1 teaspoon cumin, ground
- 1 teaspoon sweet paprika
- ½ teaspoon ancho chili powder
- 1 teaspoon onion powder

For the salsa:
- 1 small red onion, chopped
- 1 avocado, pitted, peeled and chopped
- 2 tablespoons cilantro, chopped
- Juice of 2 limes
- Salt and black pepper to the taste

Directions:
In a bowl, mix salt, pepper, chili powder, onion powder, paprika and cumin. Rub salmon with this mix, drizzle the oil and transfer to your Crockpot. Add onion, cilantro, lime juice, salt and pepper, toss a bit, cover and cook on High for 1 hour. Divide Into small bowls and serve as an appetizer with avocado sprinkled on top.
Enjoy!

Nutrition: calories 300, fat 14, fiber 4, carbs 5, protein 20

Tuna Cakes

Preparation time: 10 minutes
Cooking time: 1 hour and 20 minutes
Servings: 12

Ingredients:
- 15 ounces canned tuna, drained and flaked
- 3 eggs
- ½ teaspoon dill, dried
- 1 teaspoon parsley, dried
- ½ cup red onion, chopped
- 1 teaspoon garlic powder
- Salt and black pepper to the taste
- ½ cup tomato sauce
- A drizzle of olive oil

Directions:
In a bowl, mix tuna with salt, pepper, dill, parsley, onion, garlic powder and eggs, stir well, shape your cakes, transfer to your Crockpot after you've greased it with some oil, add tomato sauce, cover and cook on High for 1 hour and 20 minutes. Arrange on a platter and serve as an appetizer.
Enjoy!

Nutrition: calories 140, fat 2, fiber 1, carbs 6, protein 6

Creole Shrimp Appetizer

Preparation time: 10 minutes
Cooking time: 1 hour
Servings: 2

Ingredients:
- ½ pound big shrimp, peeled and deveined
- 2 teaspoons soy sauce
- 2 teaspoons olive oil
- 1 cup chicken stock
- Juice of 1 lemon
- Salt and black pepper to the taste
- 1 teaspoon Creole seasoning

Directions:
Grease your Crockpot with oil, add shrimp, soy sauce, stock, lemon juice, salt, pepper and Creole seasoning, cover and cook on High for 1 hour. Arrange shrimp on a platter and serve.
Enjoy!

Nutrition: calories 120, fat 3, fiber 1, carbs 2, protein 6

Octopus Salad

Preparation time: 10 minutes
Cooking time: 5 hours
Servings: 2

Ingredients:
- 21 ounces octopus, rinsed
- Juice of 1 lemon
- 4 celery stalks, chopped
- 3 ounces olive oil
- Salt and black pepper to the taste
- 4 tablespoons parsley, chopped

Directions:
Put the octopus your Crockpot, add water to cover, salt and pepper, cover and cook on Low for 5 hours. Drain octopus, chop, put In a salad bowl, add lemon juice, celery, oil, salt, pepper and parsley, toss and serve as an appetizer.
Enjoy!

Nutrition: calories 140, fat 10, fiber 3, carbs 6, protein 13

Cod Appetizer Salad

Preparation time: 2 hours and 10 minutes
Cooking time: 3 hours
Servings: 8

Ingredients:
- 2 cups jarred pimiento peppers, chopped
- 2 pounds salt cod
- 1 cup parsley, chopped
- 1 cup kalamata olives, pitted and chopped
- 6 tablespoons capers
- ¾ cup olive oil
- Salt and black pepper to the taste
- Juice of 2 lemons
- 4 garlic cloves, minced
- 2 celery ribs, chopped
- ½ teaspoon red chili flakes
- 1 lettuce head, leaves separated

Directions:
Put cod In your Crockpot, add water to cover, cook on Low for 3 hours, drain and transfer to a salad bowl. Add pimiento peppers, parsley, olives, capers, celery, garlic, lemon juice, salt, pepper, olive oil and chili flakes and toss to coat. Arrange lettuce leaves on a platter, add the cod salad and serve.
Enjoy!

Nutrition: calories 240, fat 4, fiber 2, carbs 6, protein 9

Hot Salmon Bites

Preparation time: 10 minutes
Cooking time: 2 hours and 10 minutes
Servings: 6

Ingredients:
- 1 and ¼ cups coconut, desiccated and unsweetened
- 1 pound salmon, cubed
- 1 egg
- Salt and black pepper
- 1 tablespoon water
- 1/3 cup coconut flour
- 3 tablespoons coconut oil
- ¼ teaspoon agar agar
- 3 garlic cloves, chopped
- ¾ cup water
- 4 Thai red chilies, chopped
- ¼ cup balsamic vinegar
- ½ cup stevia
- A pinch of salt

For the sauce:

Directions:
In a bowl, mix flour with salt and pepper and stir. In another bowl, whisk egg and 1 tablespoon water. Put the coconut In a third bowl. Dip salmon cubes In flour, egg and then In coconut and place them on a plate. Heat up a pan with the coconut oil over medium- high heat, add salmon bites, cook for 3 minutes on each side and transfer them to a plate. In your Crockpot, mix ¾ cup water with red chilies, garlic, agar agar, vinegar, stevia and salt, stir, add salmon bites, cover and cook on High for 2 hours. Arrange salmon biter on a platter and serve.
Enjoy!

Nutrition: calories 100, fat 2, fiber 4, carbs 7, protein 12

Salmon Salad

Preparation time: 10 minutes
Cooking time: 1 hour
Servings: 2

Ingredients:
- 2 medium salmon fillets
- ½ cup seafood stock
- Salt and black pepper to the taste
- A drizzle of olive oil
- 1 shallot, chopped
- 1 lettuce head, leaves torn
- 1 tablespoon lemon juice
- ¼ cup olive oil
- 2 tablespoons parsley, finely chopped

Directions:
Brush salmon fillets with a drizzle of olive oil, sprinkle with salt and pepper, put them In your Crockpot, add stock, cover and cook on High for 1 hour. Meanwhile, put shallot In a bowl, add 1 tablespoon lemon juice, salt and pepper, stir and leave aside for 10 minutes. Flake salmon, put In a bowl, add lettuce leaves, shallot, the rest of the oil and parsley, toss and serve as an appetizer.
Enjoy!

Nutrition: calories 200, fat 10, fiber 1, carbs 5, protein 16

Chili Dip

Preparation time: 10 minutes
Cooking time: 2 hours
Servings: 8

Ingredients:
- 5 ancho chilies, dried and chopped
- 2 garlic cloves, minced
- Slat and black pepper to the taste
- 1 and ½ cups water
- 2 tablespoons balsamic vinegar
- 1 and ½ teaspoons stevia
- 1 tablespoon oregano, chopped
- ½ teaspoon cumin, ground

Directions:
In your Crockpot mix water chilies, garlic, salt, pepper, stevia, cumin and oregano, stir, cover and cook on High for 2 hours. Blend using an immersion blender, add vinegar, stir, divide between bowls and serve as a snack.
Enjoy!

Nutrition: calories 85, fat 1, fiber 1, carbs 2, protein 2

Radish Dip

Preparation time: 10 minutes
Cooking time: 3 hours
Servings: 8

Ingredients:
- 1 yellow onion, chopped
- 2 tablespoons olive oil
- 5 celery ribs
- 8 garlic cloves, minced
- 4 oz radish, chopped
- 1 butternut squash, peeled and chopped
- 1 cup veggie stock
- ¼ cup lemon juice
- 1 bunch basil, chopped
- 2 bay leaves
- Salt and black pepper to the taste

Directions:
Grease your Crockpot with the oil, add celery, onions, radish, squash, garlic, stock, lemon juice, basil, bay leaves, salt and pepper, stir, cover and cook on High for 3 hours. Discard bay leaves, blend using an immersion blender, divide between bowls and serve.
Enjoy!

Nutrition: calories 143, fat 1, fiber 3, carbs 4, protein 3

Strawberry Dip

Preparation time: 10 minutes
Cooking time: 1 hour and 20 minutes
Servings: 4

Ingredients:
- 1 shallot, chopped
- 1 tablespoon coconut oil
- ¼ teaspoon cardamom powder
- 2 tablespoons ginger, minced
- ½ teaspoon cinnamon powder
- 5 oz strawberries, chopped
- 2 red hot chilies, chopped
- 1 apple, cored and chopped
- 5 tablespoons stevia
- 1 and ¼ tablespoon balsamic vinegar

Directions:
Grease your Crockpot with the oil, shallot, ginger, cinnamon, hot peppers, cardamom, strawberries, apple, stevia and vinegar, stir, cover and cook on High for 1 hour and 20 minutes Transfer to bowls and serve cold. Enjoy!

Nutrition: calories 100, fat 2, fiber 1, carbs 3, protein 1

Balsamic Mushrooms Dip

Preparation time: 10 minutes
Cooking time: 2 hours
Servings: 4

Ingredients:
- 6 ounces mushrooms, chopped
- 3 tablespoon olive oil
- 1 tablespoon thyme, chopped
- 1 garlic clove, minced
- 4 ounces beef stock
- 1 tablespoon balsamic vinegar
- 1 tablespoon mustard
- 2 tablespoon coconut cream
- 2 tablespoons parsley, finely chopped

Directions:
Grease your Crockpot with the oil, add thyme, mushrooms, garlic, vinegar, stock, mustard, coconut cream and parsley, stir, cover and cook on High for 2 hours. Stir really well, divide between bowls and serve as a snack.
Enjoy!

Nutrition: calories 140, fat 3, fiber 2, carbs 4, protein 3

Clams and Mussels Appetizer Salad

Preparation time: 10 minutes
Cooking time: 2 hours
Servings: 4

Ingredients:
- 15 small clams
- 30 mussels, scrubbed
- 2 chorizo links, sliced
- 1 yellow onion, chopped
- 10 ounces veggie stock
- 2 tablespoons parsley, chopped
- 1 teaspoon olive oil
- Lemon wedges for serving

Directions:
Grease your Crockpot with the oil and add onion and chorizo on the bottom. Add clams, mussels, stock and parsley, toss, cover and cook on High for 2 hours. Divide Into small bowls and serve with lemon wedges on the side.
Enjoy!

Nutrition: calories 172, fat 4, fiber 3, carbs 7, protein 12

Easy Clams Delight

Preparation time: 10 minutes
Cooking time: 1 hour and 20 minutes
Servings: 4

Ingredients:
- 24 clams, shucked
- 3 garlic cloves, minced
- 2 tablespoons coconut oil
- ¼ cup parsley, chopped
- ¼ cup parmesan cheese, grated
- 1 teaspoon oregano, dried
- 1 cup almonds, crushed
- 1 and ½ cups seafood stock
- Lemon wedges

Directions:
In a bowl, mix almonds with parmesan, oregano, parsley, coconut oil and garlic, stir and divide this Into exposed clams. Add the stock to your Crockpot, add clams Inside, cover and cook on High 1 hour and 20 minutes. Arrange clams on a platter and serve them as an appetizer with lemon wedges on the side.
Enjoy!

Nutrition: calories 92, fat 3, fiber 3, carbs 6, protein 5

Artichokes Appetizer

Preparation time: 10 minutes
Cooking time: 2 hours
Servings: 4

Ingredients:
- 4 big artichokes, trimmed
- Salt and black pepper to the taste
- 2 tablespoons lemon juice
- ¼ cup olive oil
- 2 teaspoons balsamic vinegar
- 1 teaspoon oregano, dried
- 2 garlic cloves, minced
- 1 cup chicken stock

Directions:
In your Crockpot, mix stock with oil, vinegar, oregano, garlic, lemon juice, salt and pepper and whisk. Add artichokes, toss a bit, cover and cook on High for 2 hours. Arrange artichokes on a platter and serve as an appetizer.
Enjoy!

Nutrition: calories 162, fat 4, fiber 2, carbs 3, protein 5

Endives Appetizer Salad

Preparation time: 10 minutes
Cooking time: 3 hours
Servings: 4

Ingredients:
- 4 endives, trimmed
- 1 cup chicken stock
- Salt and black pepper to the taste
- 2 tablespoons coconut oil
- 4 slices ham, roughly chopped
- ½ teaspoon nutmeg, ground
- 14 ounces coconut cream

Directions:
In your Crockpot, mix endives with stock, salt, pepper, oil, ham, nutmeg and coconut cream, cover and cook on High for 3 hours. Divide Into small bowls and serve as an appetizer.
Enjoy!

Nutrition: calories 152, fat 3, fiber 3, carbs 6, protein 12

Dessert Recipes

Cocoa Pudding

Preparation time: 10 minutes
Cooking time: 1 hour
Servings: 2

Ingredients:
- 2 tablespoons water
- 2 tablespoon gelatin
- 4 tablespoons stevia
- 4 tablespoons cocoa powder
- 2 cups coconut milk, hot

Directions:
In a bowl, mix milk with stevia and cocoa powder and stir well. In a bowl, mix gelatin with water, stir well, add to the cocoa mix, stir and transfer to your Crockpot. Cover, cook on High for 1 hours, divide between bowls and keep In the fridge until you serve it.
Enjoy!

Nutrition: calories 120, fat 2, fiber 1, carbs 4, protein 3

Raspberry Bars

Preparation time: 10 minutes
Cooking time: 1 hour
Servings: 12

Ingredients:
- ½ cup coconut butter
- ½ cup coconut oil
- ½ cup coconut, unsweetened and shredded
- 1 cup raspberries
- 3 tablespoons stevia

Directions:
In your Crockpot, mix coconut butter with coconut oil, coconut, raspberries and stevia, toss, cover and cook on High for 1 hour. Spread on a lined baking sheet, keep In the fridge for a few hours, slice and serve.
Enjoy!

Nutrition: calories 174, fat 5, fiber 2, carbs 4, protein 7

Mascarpone and Berries Cream

Preparation time: 10 minutes
Cooking time: 1 hour
Servings: 12

Ingredients:
- 8 ounces mascarpone cheese
- ¾ teaspoon stevia
- 1 cup coconut cream
- ½ pint blueberries
- ½ pint strawberries

Directions:
In your Crockpot, mix cream with stevia, mascarpone, blueberries and strawberries, stir, cover and cook on Low for 1 hour. Divide Into small dessert bowls and serve cold.
Enjoy!

Nutrition: calories 183, fat 4, fiber 1, carbs 3, protein 1

Simple Lemon Cake

Preparation time: 10 minutes
Cooking time: 4 hours
Servings: 12

Ingredients:
- 6 eggs
- 1 lemon, peeled and cut into quarters
- 1 teaspoon vanilla extract
- Cooking spray
- 1 teaspoon baking powder
- 9 ounces almond meal
- 2 tablespoons orange zest, grated
- 2 ounces stevia
- 4 ounces cream cheese
- 4 ounces coconut cream

Directions:
In your food processor, mix lemon with almond meal, eggs, stevia, baking powder and vanilla extract, pulse well and transfer to your Crockpot after you've greased it with cooking spray and lined with parchment paper. Cook on High for 4 hours and transfer cake to a cake plate. In a bowl, mix cream cheese with orange zest, coconut cream and stevia and stir well. Spread this well over cake, slice and serve it.
Enjoy!

Nutrition: calories 170, fat 13, fiber 2, carbs 4, protein 4

Berry Pudding

Preparation time: 10 minutes
Cooking time: 1 hour
Servings: 4

Ingredients:
- 3 tablespoons cocoa powder
- 14 ounces coconut cream
- 1 cup blackberries
- 1 cup raspberries
- 2 tablespoons stevia

Directions:
In your Crockpot, mix cream with cocoa, stevia, blackberries and raspberries, stir, cover and cook on High for 1 hour. Divide Into dessert cups and serve cold.
Enjoy!

Nutrition: calories 145, fat 4, fiber 2, carbs 6, protein 2

Stewed Raspberries

Preparation time: 10 minutes
Cooking time: 1 hour and 30 minutes
Servings: 6

Ingredients:
- 4 tablespoons stevia
- 3 cups raspberries
- 3 tablespoons natural apple juice
- 2 teaspoons lemon zest, grated

Directions:
In your Crockpot, mix raspberries with sugar, apple juice and lemon zest, stir, cover and cook at High for 1 hour and 30 minutes. Divide into small cups and serve cold.
Enjoy!

Nutrition: calories 100, fat 2, fiber 2, carbs 5, protein 5

Almond and Cocoa Cake

Preparation time: 10 minutes
Cooking time: 4 hours
Servings: 4

Ingredients:
- ½ teaspoon almond extract
- 1 cup coconut flour
- ½ cup cocoa powder
- Cooking spray
- 4 tablespoons stevia
- 3 tablespoons olive oil
- 3 eggs
- 2 teaspoons baking powder
- ½ cup almonds, sliced

Directions:
In a bowl, mix cocoa powder, almond extract, flour, eggs, stevia, oil, baking powder and almonds, whisk well and pour everything Into your Crockpot after you've greased it with cooking spray. Cover, cook on High for 4 hours, leave aside to cool down, slice, divide between plates and serve.
Enjoy!

Nutrition: calories 202, fat 4, fiber 2, carbs 8, protein 3

Pumpkin and Cauliflower Pudding

Preparation time: 30 minutes
Cooking time: 3 hours
Servings: 6

Ingredients:
- 1 cup cauliflower rice
- ½ cup water
- 3 cups coconut milk
- ½ cup dates, chopped
- 1 teaspoon cinnamon powder
- 1 cup pumpkin puree
- 4 tablespoons stevia
- 1 teaspoon vanilla extract

Directions:
Put cauliflower rice In your Crockpot, add water, milk, dates, stevia, vanilla, pumpkin and cinnamon, stir, cover and cook on High for 3 hours. Divide pudding Into bowls and serve.
Enjoy!

Nutrition: calories 120, fat 3, fiber 3, carbs 8, protein 5

Berries Marmalade

Preparation time: 10 minutes
Cooking time: 2 hours and 30 minutes
Servings: 20

Ingredients:
- 1 pound cranberries
- 1 pound strawberries
- ½ pound blueberries
- 3.5 ounces black currant
- Stevia to the taste
- Zest of 1 lemon, grated
- ½ cup water

Directions:
In your Crockpot, mix strawberries with cranberries, blueberries, currants, lemon zest, stevia and water, stir, cover and cook on High for 2 hours and 30 minutes. Divide Into dessert cups and serve cold.
Enjoy!

Nutrition: calories 100, fat 0, fiber 1, carbs 7, protein 3

Zucchini Cake

Preparation time: 10 minutes
Cooking time: 4 hours
Servings: 6

Ingredients:
- 1 cup natural applesauce
- 3 eggs, whisked
- 1 tablespoon vanilla extract
- 4 tablespoons stevia
- 2 cups zucchini, grated
- 2 and ½ cups coconut flour
- ½ cup baking cocoa powder
- 1 teaspoon baking soda
- ¼ teaspoon baking powder
- 1 teaspoon cinnamon powder
- ½ cup walnuts, chopped
- Cooking spray

Directions:
Grease your Crockpot with cooking spray, add zucchini, stevia, vanilla, eggs, applesauce, flour, cocoa powder, baking soda, baking powder, cinnamon and walnuts, whisk well, cover and cook on High for 4 hours. Leave the cake to cool down, slice and serve.
Enjoy!

Nutrition: calories 192, fat 3, fiber 6, carbs 8, protein 3

Squash Dessert

Preparation time: 10 minutes
Cooking time: 1 hour
Servings: 4

Ingredients:
- 1 tablespoon stevia
- 2 cups summer squash
- 1 tablespoon ghee, melted
- ½ cup water

Directions:
In your Crockpot, mix summer squash with stevia, ghee and water, stir, cover and cook on High for 1 hour. Divide Into dessert cups and serve them cold.
Enjoy!

Nutrition: calories 120, fat 1, fiber 1, carbs 2, protein 2

Pear Pudding

Preparation time: 5 minutes
Cooking time: 1 hour
Servings: 4

Ingredients:
- 2 cups pears, chopped
- 2 cups coconut milk
- 1 tablespoon ghee, melted
- 3 tablespoons stevia
- ½ teaspoon cinnamon powder
- 1 cup coconut flakes
- ½ cup walnuts, chopped

Directions:
In your Crockpot, mix milk with stevia, ghee, coconut, cinnamon, pears and walnuts, stir, cover and cook on High for 1 hour. Divide between bowls and serve cold.
Enjoy!

Nutrition: calories 172, fat 3, fiber 4, carbs 8, protein 7

Coconut Bars

Preparation time: 10 minutes
Cooking time: 1 hour
Servings: 10

Ingredients:
- ½ cup coconut butter
- ½ cup coconut oil
- ½ cup raspberries, dried
- ¼ cup stevia
- ½ cup coconut, shredded

Directions:
In your food processor, blend dried berries very well, transfer to your Crockpot, add coconut butter, coconut oil, stevia and coconut, stir really well, cover and cook on High for 1 hour. Transfer to a lined baking sheet, keep In the fridge for a few hours, slice and serve.
Enjoy!

Nutrition: calories 234, fat 12, fiber 2, carbs 4, protein 2

Berries and Cream Dessert

Preparation time: 10 minutes
Cooking time: 1 hour
Servings: 4

Ingredients:
- 3 tablespoons cocoa powder
- 14 ounces coconut cream
- 1 cup blackberries
- 1 cup raspberries
- 2 tablespoons stevia

Directions:
In your Crockpot, whisk cocoa powder with stevia, cream, blackberries and raspberries, cover, cook on High for 1 hour, divide Into dessert cups and serve cold.
Enjoy!

Nutrition: calories 205, fat 34, fiber 2, carbs 6, protein 2

Almonds and Coconut Granola

Preparation time: 10 minutes
Cooking time: 3 hours
Servings: 4

Ingredients:
- 1 cup coconut, unsweetened and shredded
- 1 cup almonds, chopped
- 2 tablespoons stevia
- ½ cup pumpkin seeds
- ½ cup sunflower seeds
- 3 tablespoons coconut oil
- 1 teaspoon nutmeg, ground
- 1 teaspoon apple pie spice mix

Directions:
In a bowl, mix almonds with pumpkin seeds, sunflower seeds, coconut, nutmeg and apple pie spice mix and stir well. Grease your Crockpot with the oil, add stevia and almond mix, whisk, spread well Into the pot, cover and cook on High for 3 hours. Transfer the mix to a lined baking sheet, spread well, leave aside to cool down, slice and serve.
Enjoy!

Nutrition: calories 120, fat 2, fiber 2, carbs 4, protein 5

Cherry Marmalade

Preparation time: 10 minutes
Cooking time: 3 hours
Servings: 6

Ingredients:
- 2 tablespoons lemon juice
- 3 tablespoons gelatin
- 4 cups cherries, pitted
- 3 tablespoons stevia

Directions:
In your Crockpot, mix lemon juice with gelatin, cherries and stevia, stir, cover and cook on High for 3 hours. Divide Into cups and serve cold.
Enjoy!

Nutrition: calories 211, fat 3, fiber 1, carbs 3, protein 3

Simple Cauliflower Pudding

Preparation time: 10 minutes
Cooking time: 5 hours
Servings: 4

Ingredients:
- 2 and ½ cups water
- 3 tablespoons stevia
- 2 cups cauliflower rice
- 2 cinnamon sticks
- ½ cup coconut, shredded

Directions:
In your Crockpot, mix water with stevia, cauliflower rice, cinnamon and coconut, stir, cover and cook on High for 5 hours. Divide pudding Into cups and serve cold.
Enjoy!

Nutrition: calories 113, fat 4, fiber 6, carbs 9, protein 4

Pumpkin Cake

Preparation time: 10 minutes
Cooking time: 2 hours and 20 minutes
Servings: 10

Ingredients:
- 1 and ½ teaspoons baking powder
- Cooking spray
- 1 cup pumpkin puree
- 2 cups almond flour
- ½ teaspoon baking soda
- 1 and ½ teaspoons cinnamon powder
- ¼ teaspoon ginger, ground
- 1 tablespoon coconut oil, melted
- 1 tablespoon flax meal
- 1 tablespoon vanilla extract
- 1/3 cup sugar-free maple syrup
- 1 teaspoon lemon juice

Directions:
In a bowl, flour with baking powder, baking soda, cinnamon, ginger, flaxseed, oil, vanilla, pumpkin puree, sugar-free maple syrup and lemon juice and whisk well. Grease your Crockpot with cooking spray, pour cake mix, cover and cook on Low for 2 hours and 20 minutes. Leave the cake to cool down, slice and serve.
Enjoy!

Nutrition: calories 182, fat 3, fiber 2, carbs 3, protein 1

Strawberries and Blueberries Marmalade

Preparation time: 10 minutes
Cooking time: 4 hours
Servings: 15

Ingredients:
- 14 ounces strawberries, chopped
- 20 ounces blueberries
- ½ cup stevia
- Zest of 1 lemon, grated
- 3 ounces water

Directions:
In your Crockpot, mix strawberries with stevia, lemon zest, and water, stir, cover and cook on High for 4 hours. Divide Into small jars and serve cold.
Enjoy!

Nutrition: calories 100, fat 3, fiber 2, carbs 2, protein 1

Lemon Marmalade

Preparation time: 10 minutes
Cooking time: 3 hours
Servings: 20

Ingredients:
- 2 pounds lemons, washed, peeled and sliced
- 1 cup stevia
- 1 tablespoon white vinegar

Directions:
In your Crockpot, mix lemons with stevia and vinegar, stir, cover and cook on High for 3 hours. Divide Into jars and serve cold.
Enjoy!

Nutrition: calories 100, fat 0, fiber 2, carbs 7, protein 4

Sour Apples Jam

Preparation time: 10 minutes
Cooking time: 5 hours
Servings: 20

Ingredients:
- 2 pounds apples, washed, peeled and sliced
- 1 cup stevia
- 1 tablespoon cinnamon powder

Directions:
In your Crockpot, mix apples with stevia and cinnamon, stir, cover and cook on Low for 5 hours. Divide between bowls and serve cold.
Enjoy!

Nutrition: calories 100, fat 0, fiber 2, carbs 7, protein 4

Rhubarb and Berries Marmalade

Preparation time: 10 minutes
Cooking time: 3 hours
Servings: 25

Ingredients:
- 1/3 cup water
- 2 pounds rhubarb, chopped
- 2 pounds blueberries, chopped
- 4 tablespoons stevia
- 1 tablespoon mint, chopped

Directions:
In your Crockpot, mix water with rhubarb, berries, stevia and mint, stir, cover and cook on High for 3 hours. Divide Into cups and serve cold.
Enjoy!

Nutrition: calories 100, fat 1, fiber 4, carbs 10, protein 2

Sweet Plums

Preparation time: 10 minutes
Cooking time: 3 hours
Servings: 10

Ingredients:
- 14 plums, pitted and halved
- 4 tablespoons stevia
- 1 teaspoon cinnamon powder
- ¼ cup water

Directions:
In your Crockpot, mix plums with stevia, cinnamon and water, stir, cover, cook on Low for 3 hours, divide Into cups and serve cold.
Enjoy!

Nutrition: calories 150, fat 2, fiber 1, carbs 2, protein 3

Fruit Bowls

Preparation time: 10 minutes
Cooking time: 2 hours
Servings: 10

Ingredients:
- 3 pears, cored and chopped
- 2 cups sour apples
- 1 teaspoon ginger powder
- ¼ cup erythritol
- 1 teaspoon lemon juice
- 1 teaspoon lemon zest, grated

Directions:
In your Crockpot, mix pears with apples, ginger, erythritol, lemon juice and lemon zest, stir, cover, cook on High for 2 hours, divide between bowls and serve cold.
Enjoy!

Nutrition: calories 140, fat 3, fiber 4, carbs 6, protein 6

Sweet Strawberry Cream

Preparation time: 10 minutes
Cooking time: 3 hours
Servings: 15

Ingredients:
- 2 tablespoons lemon juice
- 2 pounds strawberries, chopped
- ½ cup stevia
- 1 teaspoon cinnamon powder
- 1 teaspoon vanilla extract

Directions:
In your Crockpot, mix strawberries with stevia, lemon juice, cinnamon and vanilla, cover and cook on Low for 3 hours. Blend a bit using your immersion blender, divide between bowls and keep In the fridge until you serve it.
Enjoy!

Nutrition: calories 100, fat 0, fiber 1, carbs 2, protein 2

Sour Apple Stew

Preparation time: 10 minutes
Cooking time: 4 hours
Servings: 6

Ingredients:
- 6 apples, cored, peeled and sliced
- 1 and ½ cups almond flour
- Cooking spray
- 3 tablespoons stevia
- 1 tablespoon cinnamon powder
- ¾ cup cashew butter, melted

Directions:
Grease your Crockpot with cooking spray, add apples, flour, stevia, cinnamon and coconut butter, stir gently, cover, cook on High for 4 hours, divide between bowls and serve cold.
Enjoy!

Nutrition: calories 180, fat 5, fiber 5, carbs 8, protein 4

Berry Pie

Preparation time: 10 minutes
Cooking time: 2 hours
Servings: 6

Ingredients:
- 1 pound fresh blackberries
- 1 pound fresh blueberries
- ¾ cup water
- 5 tablespoons stevia
- 1 cup almond flour
- ½ cup arrowroot powder
- 1 teaspoon baking powder
- 1/3 cup coconut milk
- 1 egg, whisked
- 1 teaspoon lemon zest, grated
- 3 tablespoons coconut oil, melted

Directions:
In your Crockpot, mix blueberries, blackberries, stevia, water and half of the almond flour, cover and cook on High for 1 hour. Meanwhile, In a bowl, mix the rest of the flour with arrowroot, and baking powder and stir well. Add egg, milk, oil and lemon zest, stir, drop spoonfuls of this mix over the berries from the Crockpot, cover and cook on High for 1 more hour. Leave pie aside to cool down, divide into dessert bowls and serve.
Enjoy!

Nutrition: calories 240, fat 4, fiber 3, carbs 6, protein 6

Simple Lemon Pudding

Preparation time: 10 minutes
Cooking time: 5 hours
Servings: 4

Ingredients:
- Cooking spray
- 1 teaspoon baking powder
- 1 cup almond flour
- 1/3 cup erythritol
- ½ teaspoon cinnamon, ground
- 3 tablespoons coconut oil, melted
- ½ cup almond milk
- ½ cup pecans, chopped
- ¾ cup water
- ½ cup lemon peel, grated
- ¾ cup lemon juice

Directions:
In a bowl, mix flour with half of the erythritol, baking powder and cinnamon and stir. Add 2 tablespoons oil, milk, pecans, stir and pour this Into Crockpot after you've greased it with cooking spray. Heat up a small pan over medium- high heat, add water, lemon juice, lemon peel, the rest of the oil and the rest of the erythritol, stir, bring to a simmer, pour over the mix In the Crockpot, cover and cook on Low for 5 hours. Divide Into dessert bowls and serve.
Enjoy!

Nutrition: calories 182, fat 3, fiber 1, carbs 8, protein 6

Stuffed Apples

Preparation time: 10 minutes
Cooking time: 2 hours
Servings: 4

Ingredients:
- 4 apples, tops cut off and cored
- 4 figs
- 2 tablespoons stevia
- 1 teaspoon ginger powder
- ¼ cup pecans, chopped
- 2 teaspoons lemon zest, grated
- ¼ teaspoon nutmeg, ground
- ½ teaspoon cinnamon powder
- 1 tablespoon lemon juice
- 1 tablespoon coconut oil
- ½ cup water

Directions:
In a bowl, mix figs with stevia, ginger, pecans, lemon zest, nutmeg, cinnamon, oil and lemon juice, whisk really well and stuff your apples with this mix. Put the water In your Crockpot, arrange apples, cover, cook on High for 2 hours, divide on dessert plates and serve.
Enjoy!

Nutrition: calories 200, fat 1, fiber 2, carbs 4, protein 7

Chocolate Cake

Preparation time: 10 minutes
Cooking time: 3 hours
Servings: 10

Ingredients:
- 1 cup almond flour
- ½ cup cocoa powder
- 3 tablespoons swerve
- 1 and ½ teaspoons baking powder
- 3 eggs
- Cooking spray
- 4 tablespoons coconut oil, melted
- ¾ teaspoon vanilla extract
- 2/3 cup almond milk
- 1/3 cup keto chocolate chips

Directions:
In a bowl, mix swerve with almond flour, cocoa powder, baking powder, milk, oil, eggs, chocolate chips and vanilla extract, whisk really well, pour this Into your lined and greased Crockpot and cook on Low for 3 hours. Leave the cake aside to cool down, slice and serve.
Enjoy!

Nutrition: calories 200, fat 12, fiber 4, carbs 8, protein 6

Stewed Pears

Preparation time: 10 minutes
Cooking time: 4 hours
Servings: 4

Ingredients:
- 4 pears, peeled and tops cut off and cored
- 5 cardamom pods
- 2 cups water
- ½ cup sugar-free maple syrup
- 1 cinnamon stick
- 1 Inch ginger, grated

Directions:
Put the pears In your Crockpot, add cardamom pods, water, sugar-free maple syrup, cinnamon and ginger, cover and cook on Low for 4 hours. Divide between bowls and serve with the sauce drizzled on top.
Enjoy!

Nutrition: calories 200, fat 4, fiber 2, carbs 3, protein 4

Maple Pecans

Preparation time: 10 minutes
Cooking time: 1 hour
Servings: 3

Ingredients:
- 2 teaspoons vanilla extract
- 3 cups pecans
- ¼ cup sugar-free maple syrup
- 1 tablespoon coconut oil

Directions:
Put your pecans In the Crockpot, add vanilla extract, oil and sugar-free maple syrup, toss to coat and cook on High for 1 hour. Divide Into cups and serve.
Enjoy!

Nutrition: calories 200, fat 2, fiber 2, carbs 4, protein 7

Plum and Cinnamon Mousse

Preparation time: 10 minutes
Cooking time: 2 hours
Servings: 20

Ingredients:

- 4 pounds plums, stones removed and cut into medium wedges
- 1 cup water
- 2 tablespoons erythritol
- 1 teaspoon cinnamon powder

Directions:
Put plums, water, erythritol and cinnamon In your Crockpot, cover and cook on Low for 2 hours. Divide bowls and serve cold.
Enjoy!

Nutrition: calories 103, fat 0, fiber 1, carbs 2, protein 4

Passion Fruit Dessert Cream

Preparation time: 10 minutes
Cooking time: 4 hours
Servings: 6

Ingredients:

- 1 cup water
- 4 passion fruits, pulp and seeds separated
- 3 and ½ ounces sugar-free maple syrup
- 3 eggs
- 2 ounces coconut oil, melted
- 3 and ½ ounces coconut milk
- ½ cup almond flour
- ½ teaspoon baking powder

Directions:
In your Crockpot, mix water with passion fruits pulp and seeds, sugar-free maple syrup, eggs, coconut, almond milk, almond flour and baking powder, whisk really well, cover and cook on Low for 4 hours. Whisk really well, divide between bowls and serve cold.
Enjoy!

Nutrition: calories 230, fat 12, fiber 3, carbs 7, protein 8

Cherry and Cocoa Mousse

Preparation time: 10 minutes
Cooking time: 4 hours
Servings: 10

Ingredients:
- ½ cup dark cocoa powder
- 3 cups water
- ¼ cup sugar-free maple syrup
- 1 pound cherries, pitted and halved
- 2 tablespoons stevia

Directions:
In your Crockpot, mix cocoa powder with water, sugar-free maple syrup, cherries, and stevia, stir, cover and cook on Low for 4 hours. Divide between bowls and serve cold.
Enjoy!

Nutrition: calories 207, fat 1, fiber 4, carbs 5, protein 2

Grapefruit and Mint Sauce

Preparation time: 10 minutes
Cooking time: 4 hours
Servings: 3

Ingredients:
- 1 cup water
- ½ cup sugar-free maple syrup
- ½ cup mint, chopped
- 2 grapefruits, peeled and chopped

Directions:
In your Crockpot, mix grapefruit with water, sugar-free maple syrup, and mint, stir, cover and cook on Low for 4 hours. Divide between bowls and serve cold.
Enjoy!

Nutrition: calories 120, fat 1, fiber, 2, carbs 2, protein 1

Maple Figs Stew

Preparation time: 10 minutes
Cooking time: 1 hour
Servings: 4

Ingredients:
- 2 tablespoons coconut butter
- 6 figs, halved
- 1 cup almonds, chopped
- ¼ cup sugar-free maple syrup

Directions:
In your Crockpot, mix coconut butter with sugar-free maple syrup, whisk well, add figs and almonds, toss, cover and cook on Low for 1 hour. Divide between bowls and serve right away.
Enjoy!

Nutrition: calories 170, fat 6, fiber 5, carbs 6, protein 8

Special Apple Cake

Preparation time: 10 minutes
Cooking time: 2 hours and 30 minutes
Servings: 6

Ingredients:
- 3 cups apples, cored and cubed
- 1/3 cup swerve
- 1 tablespoon vanilla
- 2 eggs
- 1 tablespoon pumpkin pie spice
- 2 cups almond flour
- 1 tablespoon baking powder
- 1 tablespoon ghee, melted

Directions:
In your Crockpot, mix apples with swerve, vanilla, eggs, apple pie spice, almond flour, baking powder and ghee, cover and cook on High for 2 hours and 20 minutes. Leave the special cake to cool down, slice and serve.
Enjoy!

Nutrition: calories 170, fat 2, fiber 4, carbs 12, protein 4

Vanilla Espresso Cream

Preparation time: 10 minutes
Cooking time: 1 hour and 30 minutes
Servings: 4

Ingredients:
- 1 cup coconut milk
- 1 cup hemp hearts
- 2 and ½ cups water
- ½ tablespoon stevia
- 1 teaspoon espresso powder
- 2 teaspoons vanilla extract

Directions:
In your Crockpot, mix hemp with water, stevia, milk and espresso powder, stir, cover and cook on High for 1 hour and 30 minutes Add vanilla extract, stir, divide between bowls and serve cold
Enjoy!

Nutrition: calories 200, fat 4, fiber 6, carbs 12, protein 4

Lemon and Blackberries Cream

Preparation time: 30 minutes
Cooking time: 1 hour
Servings: 4

Ingredients:
- 1 cup coconut milk
- Zest of 1 lemon, grated
- 6 egg yolks
- 1 cup coconut cream
- 1 cup water
- 3 tablespoons stevia
- ½ cup fresh blackberries

Directions:
In your Crockpot, mix coconut milk with lemon zest, whisked egg yolks, cream, water, stevia and blackberries, toss, cover and cook on High for 1 hour. Divide between bowls and serve cold.
Enjoy!

Nutrition: calories 162, fat 4, fiber 6, carbs 9, protein 4

Stewed Figs

Preparation time: 10 minutes
Cooking time: 1 hour and 20 minutes
Servings: 15

Ingredients:
- 1 cup water
- 1 pound figs
- ½ cup pine nuts, toasted
- 4 tablespoons stevia

Directions:
In your Crockpot, mix figs with water, stevia and pine nuts, toss, cover and cook on High for 1 hour and 20 minutes. Divide stewed figs Into small bowls and serve them cold.
Enjoy!

Nutrition: calories 132, fat 4, fiber 3, carbs 7, protein 4

Carrot Cake

Preparation time: 10 minutes
Cooking time: 4 hours
Servings: 4

Ingredients:
- 5 ounces almond flour
- ¾ teaspoon baking powder
- ½ teaspoon baking soda
- ½ teaspoon cinnamon powder
- ¼ teaspoon nutmeg, ground
- ½ teaspoon allspice
- 1 egg
- 3 tablespoons coconut cream
- 2 tablespoons stevia
- ¼ cup water
- 4 tablespoons coconut oil, melted
- ½ cup carrots, grated
- 1/3 cup pecans, toasted and chopped
- 1/3 cup coconut flakes
- Cooking spray

Directions:
In a bowl, mix flour with baking soda and powder, allspice, cinnamon and nutmeg and stir. In a second bowl, mix the egg with coconut cream, stevia, water, oil, carrots, pecans and coconut flakes and stir well. Combine the two mixtures, stir very well everything, pour this Into your Crockpot after you've greased it with cooking spray, cover and cook on Low for 4 hours. Leave the cake to cool down, then cut and serve it.
Enjoy!

Nutrition: calories 251, fat 4, fiber 4, carbs 7, protein 4

Strawberry Marmalade

Preparation time: 10 minutes
Cooking time: 3 hours
Servings: 6

Ingredients:
- 4 and ½ cups strawberries
- 1 cup stevia
- 2 tablespoons ginger, grated
- ½ cup water

Directions:
In your Crockpot, mix strawberries with stevia, ginger and water, stir, cover and cook on High for 3 hours. Divide marmalade Into jars and serve as a dessert.
Enjoy!

Nutrition: calories 100, fat 0, fiber 3, carbs 6, protein 4

Raspberry Cream

Preparation time: 10 minutes
Cooking time: 2 hours
Servings: 4

Ingredients:
- 3 tablespoons stevia
- 12 ounces raspberries
- 2 egg yolks, whisked
- 2 tablespoons lemon juice
- 2 tablespoons coconut oil, melted

Directions:
In your Crockpot, mix raspberries with stevia, egg yolks, lemon juice and melted coconut oil, whisk well, cover and cook on High for 2 hours. Whisk your cream one more time, divide into small cups and serve cold.
Enjoy!

Nutrition: calories 123, fat 4, fiber 4, carbs 7, protein 3

Dried Fruits Pudding

Preparation time: 10 minutes
Cooking time: 3 hours
Servings: 4

Ingredients:
- 4 ounces dried cranberries, soaked In hot water, drained and chopped
- A drizzle of avocado oil
- 2 ounces dried apricots, chopped
- 1 cup almond flour
- 3 teaspoons baking powder
- 2 tablespoons erythritol
- 1 teaspoon ginger powder
- ½ teaspoon cinnamon powder
- 15 tablespoons ghee, melted
- 3 tablespoons sugar-free maple syrup
- 4 eggs
- ½ carrot, grated

Directions:
In a blender, mix flour with baking powder, erythritol, cinnamon, salt and ginger and pulse a few times. Add ghee, sugar-free maple syrup, eggs, dried cranberries, dried apricots and carrot, fold them Into the batter and spread this Into your Crockpot after you've greased it with a drizzle of avocado oil. Cover, cook on Low for 3 hours, leave aside to cool down, divide between bowls and serve.
Enjoy!

Nutrition: calories 271, fat 4, fiber 6, carbs 12, protein 4

Avocado Cake

Preparation time: 10 minutes
Cooking time: 4 hours
Servings: 6

Ingredients:
- 1/8 teaspoon almond extract
- 1 cup avocados, stoned and chopped
- 4 tablespoons coconut flour
- ½ cup cocoa powder
- 4 tablespoons erythritol
- 3 tablespoons avocado oil
- 3 eggs
- 2 teaspoons baking powder
- ¼ cup almonds, slice

Directions:
In a bowl, mix almond extract with avocado, flour, cocoa, erythritol, oil, eggs, baking powder and almonds, whisk well, transfer to your Crockpot after you've greased it with cooking spray, cover and cook on Low for 4 hours. Leave the cake to cool down, slice and serve.
Enjoy!

Nutrition: calories 164, fat 4, fiber 6, carbs 8, protein 4

Ricotta and Dates Cake

Preparation time: 30 minutes
Cooking time: 4 hours
Servings: 6

Ingredients:
- 1 pound ricotta
- 2 oz dates, soaked for 15 minutes and drained
- 2 tablespoons erythritol
- 4 eggs
- ½ teaspoon vanilla extract
- Zest of ½ lemon, grated
- Cooking spray

Directions:
In a bowl, whisk ricotta until it softens. Add eggs, erythritol, dates, vanilla and lemon zest, whisk well, pour Into your Crockpot after you've greased it with cooking spray, cover and cook on Low for 4 hours. Leave the cake to cool down, slice and serve.
Enjoy!

Nutrition: calories 200, fat 6, fiber 6, carbs 8, protein 10

Rhubarb Mousse

Preparation time: 10 minutes
Cooking time: 3 hours
Servings: 10

Ingredients:
- 1 cup water
- 2 pounds rhubarb, chopped
- 2 tablespoon stevia
- 1/3 pound strawberries, chopped

Directions:
Put rhubarb, water, stevia and strawberries In your Crockpot, cover and cook on High for 3 hours. Divide between bowls and serve cold.
Enjoy!

Nutrition: calories 100, fat 4, fiber 5, carbs 6, protein 1

Squash Pudding

Preparation time: 10 minutes
Cooking time: 4 hours
Servings: 8

Ingredients:
- Cooking spray
- 2 tablespoons stevia
- 3 eggs
- ½ cup almond flour
- ½ teaspoon allspice, ground
- ½ teaspoon cinnamon powder
- A pinch of nutmeg
- ½ teaspoon baking soda
- 2/3 cup ghee, melted
- ½ cup pecans, chopped
- 1 cup butternut squash, grated

Directions:
In a bowl, mix stevia with eggs, almond flour, allspice, cinnamon, nutmeg, baking soda, melted ghee, pecans, squash, stir well, pour Into your Crockpot after you've greased it with cooking spray, cover and cook on Low for 4 hours. Leave pudding to cool down, slice and serve.
Enjoy!

Nutrition: calories 200, fat 4, fiber 6, carbs 12, protein 4

Chestnut Cream

Preparation time: 10 minutes
Cooking time: 3 hours
Servings: 10

Ingredients:
- 4 tablespoons stevia
- 11 ounces water
- 1 and ½ pounds chestnuts, halved and peeled

Directions:
In your Crockpot, mix stevia with water and chestnuts, stir, cover and cook on Low for 3 hours. Blend using your immersion blender, divide into small cups and serve.
Enjoy!

Nutrition: calories 102, fat 1, fiber 0, carbs 5, protein 3

Conclusion

A Ketogenic diet might be exactly what you need in your life right now! This diet is easy to follow and it brings you so many health benefits!
On the other hand, slow cooker are some of the most popular kitchen appliances available on the market these days.
These wonderful tools help you cook delicious and healthy meals for all your loved ones.

Now, we ask you: what do you get from combining one of the healthiest diets with the best cooking tool?
Well, the answer is pretty simple: you get the cooking experience of a lifetime!
So, don't hesitate! Get your hands on this amazing cooking journal and start your new and improved life!
Start cooking Ketogenic style with your amazing slow cooker!
Enjoy!

Recipe Index

ALMOND FLOUR
Cod Sticks, 89
Pumpkin Cake, 117
Sour Apple Stew, 121
Berry Pie, 122
Simple Lemon Pudding, 122
Chocolate Cake, 123
Special Apple Cake, 127
Carrot Cake, 129
Dried Fruits Pudding, 131
Squash Pudding, 133

ALMOND MILK
Salmon Omelet, 17
Cauliflower Rice Pudding, 27
Maple and Cauliflower Rice Pudding, 28
Chocolate Cake, 123

ALMONDS
Simple Coconut Mix, 20
Balsamic Kale, 74
Spicy Nuts Mix, 93
Easy Clams Delight, 107
Almond and Cocoa Cake, 112
Almonds and Coconut Granola, 116
Maple Figs Stew, 127

APPLES
Sour Apples and Strawberries Breakfast Mix, 32
Cabbage and Apples Side Dish, 64
Sour Apples Jam, 119
Fruit Bowls, 120
Sour Apple Stew, 121
Stuffed Apples, 123
Special Apple Cake, 127

APRICOTS
Dried Fruits Pudding, 131

ARTICHOKES
Artichoke and Coconut Spread, 88
Artichokes Appetizer, 108

ARUGULA
Mediterranean Frittata, 12
Mushroom and Arugula Mix, 69

ASPARAGUS
Tasty Asparagus Casserole, 13
Tasty Asparagus and Mushroom Casserole, 13
Easy Asparagus, 81

AVOCADO
Cauliflower Rice Pudding and Salsa, 26
Fajita Bowls, 28
Breakfast Pork and Avocado Mix, 31
Salmon Salsa, 101
Avocado Cake, 131

BACON
Egg and Bacon Casserole, 10
Incredible Turkey and Bacon Casserole, 14
Simple Bacon and Collard Greens, 36
Delicious Bacon Chicken, 46
Bok Choy and Bacon Mix, 77
Collard Greens, Bacon and Tomatoes, 79

BEANS
Cheesy Green Beans, 66

BEEF
Beef Breakfast Bowl, 17
Beef and Bok Choy Mix, 18
Beef and Radish Breakfast, 20
Corned Beef Brisket, 38
Simple Beef Stew, 39
Spicy Curry, 39
Beef and Cabbage Stew, 40
Beef and Veggie Stew, 40
Red Curry, 41
Tasty Meatballs, 41
Simple Shredded Beef, 42
American Beef Brisket, 42
Mexican Beef Stew, 43
Indian Beef Mix, 43
Beef Tongue Mix, 44
Ground Beef Soup, 44
Simple Oxtail Stew, 49
Beef Roast Soup, 51
Beef Party Rolls, 84
Party Meatballs, 90
Beef Jerky Snack, 98

BELL PEPPERS
Healthy Veggie Casserole, 11
Bell Pepper and Olives Frittata, 24
Breakfast Veggies Mix, 30
Colored Bell Peppers Mix, 76
Bell Peppers Appetizer, 87
Mushroom and Bell Peppers Spread, 88

BLACKBERRIES
Berry Pudding, 111

Berries and Cream Dessert, 115
Berry Pie, 122
Lemon and Blackberries Cream, 128

BLUEBERRIES
Berry Butter, 26
Mascarpone and Berries Cream, 110
Berries Marmalade, 113
Strawberries and Blueberries Marmalade, 118
Rhubarb and Berries Marmalade, 119
Berry Pie, 122

BOK CHOY
Beef and Bok Choy Mix, 18
Bok Choy and Bacon Mix, 77

BROCCOLI
Creamy Eggs and Turkey Mix, 9
Yellow Chicken Curry, 47
Maple Salmon with Broccoli and Cauliflower, 55
Cauliflower and Broccoli Fresh Mix, 60
Simple Broccoli Side Dish, 75
Broccoli and Tomatoes Mix, 76

BRUSSELS SPROUTS
Eggs and Brussels Sprouts Breakfast, 21
Brussels Sprouts and Onions, 64
Brussels Sprouts and Bacon, 67

CABBAGE
Corned Beef Brisket, 38
Beef and Cabbage Stew, 40
Mexican Veggie Mix, 59
Cabbage and Apples Side Dish, 64
Napa Cabbage Mix, 68
Hungarian Cabbage Side Dish, 71
Beef Party Rolls, 84

CAPERS
Red Chard and Capers, 74

CARROTS
Carrot Cake, 129

CASHEWS
Tomatoes Casserole, 23
Simple Cashew Spread, 84
Cashew Hummus, 86
Spicy Nuts Mix, 93

CAULIFLOWER
Chorizo and Cauliflower Mix, 19
Cauliflower Rice Pudding and Salsa, 26
Cauliflower Rice Pudding, 27

Maple and Cauliflower Rice Pudding, 28
Cauliflower and Mushroom Bowls, 33
Simple Pork and Cauliflower Rice, 37
Maple Salmon with Broccoli and Cauliflower, 55
Cauliflower and Broccoli Fresh Mix, 60
Special Cauliflower Rice Mix, 61
Rustic Mashed Cauliflower, 61
Fall Veggie Mix, 63
Beef Party Rolls, 84
Squash and Cauliflower Spread, 85
Mixed Veggies Spread, 86
Bell Peppers Appetizer, 87
Spicy Cauliflower Dip, 93
Pumpkin and Cauliflower Pudding, 112
Simple Cauliflower Pudding, 117

CELERY
Beef and Veggie Stew, 40
Creamy Celery Side Dish, 77
Stewed Celery Mix, 78
Octopus Salad, 103
Radish Dip, 104

CHARD
Garlicky Swiss Chard, 69
Red Chard Mix, 70
Balsamic Swiss Chard with Pine Nuts and Raisins, 72
Balsamic Spinach and Chard, 72
Red Chard and Capers, 74
Spanish Spinach Mix, 81
Squash and Swiss Chard Mix, 82

CHEDDAR CHEESE
Tasty Spinach Quiche, 10
Egg and Bacon Casserole, 10
Breakfast Omelet, 11
Delicious Egg Scramble, 12
Tasty Asparagus Casserole, 13

CHERRIES
Cherry Marmalade, 116
Cherry and Cocoa Mousse, 126

CHESTNUTS
Chestnut Cream, 133

CHIA SEEDS
Easy Chia Pudding, 21

CHICKEN
Spinach and Feta Quiche, 15
Delicious Chicken Frittata, 22
Different Chicken Omelet, 22

Chicken Drumsticks, 45
Special Chicken Soup, 45
Delicious Slow Cooked Chicken, 46
Delicious Bacon Chicken, 46
Chicken Curry, 47
Yellow Chicken Curry, 47
Delicious Creamy Chicken, 52
Chicken Wings Appetizer, 89
Stuffed Chicken Breast Appetizer, 92
Cheesy Party Wings, 99
Chicken Rolls, 100

CHILI
Chorizo and Cauliflower Mix, 19

CHORIZO
Chorizo and Cauliflower Mix, 19

CLAMS
Clams and Mussels Appetizer Salad, 107
Easy Clams Delight, 107

COCOA POWDER
Cocoa Pudding, 109
Almond and Cocoa Cake, 112
Chocolate Cake, 123
Cherry and Cocoa Mousse, 126

COCONUT
Hot Salmon Bites, 104
Raspberry Bars, 109
Almonds and Coconut Granola, 116
Simple Cauliflower Pudding, 117

COCONUT BUTTER
Raspberry Bars, 109
Coconut Bars, 115

COCONUT CREAM
Simple Coconut Mix, 20
Easy Chia Pudding, 21
Delicious Creamy Chicken, 52
Creamy Celery Side Dish, 77
Creamy Eggplant and Tomatoes, 83
Spinach and Chestnut Dip, 87
Artichoke and Coconut Spread, 88
Coconut Crab Spread, 95
Cheese Dip, 96
Different Cream Cheese Dip, 97
Salmon Cakes, 101
Endives Appetizer Salad, 108
Berry Pudding, 111
Berries and Cream Dessert, 115
Lemon and Blackberries Cream, 128

COCONUT FLAKES
Pear Pudding, 114

COCONUT FLOUR
Almond and Cocoa Cake, 112
Zucchini Cake, 113

COCONUT MILK
Tasty Asparagus and Mushroom Casserole, 13
Turkey Casserole, 15
Pear Breakfast Bowls, 25
Butternut Squash Mix, 31
Spicy Curry, 39
Red Curry, 41
Chicken Drumsticks, 45
Chicken Curry, 47
Yellow Chicken Curry, 47
Creamy Salmon Soup, 53
Creamy Clams, 58
Rustic Mashed Cauliflower, 61
Fast and Creamy Fennel Mix, 75
Squash and Cauliflower Spread, 85
Party Meatballs, 90
Curried Shrimp Appetizer, 91
Cocoa Pudding, 109
Pumpkin and Cauliflower Pudding, 112
Pear Pudding, 114
Passion Fruit Dessert Cream, 125
Vanilla Espresso Cream, 128

CRANBERRIES
Turkey, Cranberries and Cauliflower Bowls, 33
Berries Marmalade, 113
Dried Fruits Pudding, 131

CREAM CHEESE
Cheese Dip, 96
Different Cream Cheese Dip, 97
Simple Lemon Cake, 110

CURRY
Indian Beef Mix, 43

DATES
Ricotta and Dates Cake, 132

EGGPLANTS
Eggplant and Kale Mix, 63
Creamy Eggplant and Tomatoes, 83
Eggplant and Tomato Salsa, 85
Veggie Party Mix, 94

EGGS
Delicious Breakfast Pie, 9

Creamy Eggs and Turkey Mix, 9
Egg and Bacon Casserole, 10
Breakfast Omelet, 11
Healthy Veggie Casserole, 11
Delicious Egg Scramble, 12
Italian Eggs, 14
Turkey Casserole, 15
Spicy Turkey and Eggs Mix, 16
Kale Frittata, 16
Salmon Omelet, 17
Salami and Eggs Casserole, 19
Eggs and Brussels Sprouts Breakfast, 21
Delicious Chicken Frittata, 22
Different Chicken Omelet, 22
Pork Butt and Eggs Mix, 29
Simple Lemon Cake, 110
Raspberry Cream, 130
Dried Fruits Pudding, 131

ENDIVES
Endives Appetizer Salad, 108

FENNEL
Fast and Creamy Fennel Mix, 75

FETA CHEESE
Spinach and Feta Quiche, 15
Kale Frittata, 16
Burrito Bowls, 23

FIGS
Stewed Figs, 129

FISH
Spicy Tuna Loin, 56
Cod Sticks, 89
Tuna Cakes, 102
Cod Appetizer Salad, 103

GOAT CHEESE
Mediterranean Frittata, 12
Goat Cheese and Mushrooms Casserole, 24
Bell Pepper and Olives Frittata, 24
Simple Cherry Tomatoes and Onion Mix, 82

GRAPEFRUIT
Grapefruit and Mint Compote, 126

GREENS
Simple Bacon and Collard Greens, 36
Lemony Collard Greens, 78
Collard Greens, Bacon and Tomatoes, 79
Mustard Greens and Garlic, 79
Cheesy Collard Greens, 80

Spring Green Mix, 80

HEMP
Vanilla Espresso Cream, 128

KALE
Kale Frittata, 16
Leek, Kale and Turkey Breakfast, 29
Easy Lamb Curry, 51
Eggplant and Kale Mix, 63
Kale Side Dish, 70
Balsamic Kale, 74

LAMB
Lamb Legs, 50
Easy Lamb Curry, 51
Lamb Shoulder Mix, 52

LEEK
Leek, Kale and Turkey Breakfast, 29
Thai Pompano with Leeks, 56
Braised Squid, 57

LEMON
Simple Lemon Cake, 110
Lemon Marmalade, 118
Simple Lemon Pudding, 122
Lemon and Blackberries Cream, 128

LETTUCE
Breakfast Pork Salad, 32
Salmon Salad, 104

MAPLE SYRUP
Stewed Pears, 124
Maple Pecans, 124
Maple Figs Stew, 127

MASCARPONE
Mascarpone and Berries Cream, 110

MOZZARELLA
Different Cream Cheese Dip, 97
Zucchini and Tomato Dip, 97

MUSHROOMS
Tasty Spinach Quiche, 10
Tasty Asparagus and Mushroom Casserole, 13
Beef Breakfast Bowl, 17
Goat Cheese and Mushrooms Casserole, 24
Cauliflower and Mushroom Bowls, 33
Delicious Pork Stew, 35
Tasty Pork Shanks, 36
Simple Beef Stew, 39

Fresh Veggie Side Dish, 59
Simple Mushrooms Caps Side Dish, 65
Herbed Mushrooms Mix, 66
Mushroom and Arugula Mix, 69
Mushrooms Winter Mix, 71
Mixed Veggies Spread, 86
Mushroom and Bell Peppers Spread, 88
Stuffed Mushrooms, 99
Balsamic Mushrooms Dip, 106

OKRA
Fresh Veggie Side Dish, 59
Okra and Mint, 68

OLIVES
Beef Breakfast Bowl, 17
Bell Pepper and Olives Frittata, 24
Cod Appetizer Salad, 103

PARMESAN
Cheesy Green Beans, 66
Cherry Tomatoes Side Dish, 73
Different Cream Cheese Dip, 97
Cheesy Party Wings, 99
Easy Clams Delight, 107

PARSLEY
Colored Bell Peppers Mix, 76
Stewed Celery Mix, 78
Cod Appetizer Salad, 103

PARSNIP
Squash and Parsnips Mix, 62

PASSION FRUIT
Passion Fruit Dessert Cream, 125

PEARS
Pear Breakfast Bowls, 25
Pear Pudding, 114
Fruit Bowls, 120
Stewed Pears, 124

PECANS
Pecans Snack, 90
Pecans Snack, 92
Spicy Nuts Mix, 93
Simple Lemon Pudding, 122
Maple Pecans, 124

PLUMS
Sweet Plums, 120
Plum and Cinnamon Compote, 125

POMPANO
Thai Pompano with Leeks, 56

PORK
Mexican Pork Breakfast, 18
Pork Butt and Eggs Mix, 29
Meatloaf, 30
Breakfast Pork and Avocado Mix, 31
Breakfast Pork Salad, 32
Delicious Pork Chili, 34
Spiced Pork Ribs, 34
Delicious Pork Stew, 35
Simple Kalua Pork, 35
Tasty Pork Shanks, 36
Simple Pork and Cauliflower Rice, 37
Chili Verde, 37
Tender Pork Loin, 38

PUMPKIN
Pumpkin Butter, 27
Tasty Pork Shanks, 36
Pumpkin and Cauliflower Pudding, 112
Almonds and Coconut Granola, 116
Pumpkin Cake, 117

PUMPKIN SEEDS
Walnuts and Pumpkin Seeds Snack, 94

RABBIT
Rabbit Stew, 50

RADISH
Beef and Radish Breakfast, 20
Napa Cabbage Mix, 68
Creamy Radish Mix, 83
Radish Dip, 104

RASPBERRIES
Raspberry Bars, 109
Berry Pudding, 111
Stewed Raspberries, 111
Coconut Bars, 115
Berries and Cream Dessert, 115
Raspberry Cream, 130

RHUBARB
Rhubarb and Berries Marmalade, 119
Rhubarb Mousse, 132

RICOTTA CHEESE
Zucchini and Cheese Rolls, 100
Ricotta and Dates Cake, 132

SALAMI
Salami and Eggs Casserole, 19

SALMON
Salmon Omelet, 17
Creamy Salmon Soup, 53
Seafood Chowder, 54
Maple Salmon with Broccoli and Cauliflower, 55
Salmon with Cilantro Sauce, 57
Steamed Salmon, 58
Salmon Cakes, 101
Salmon Salsa, 101
Hot Salmon Bites, 104
Salmon Salad, 104

SEAFOOD
Tasty Seafood Stew, 54
Seafood Chowder, 54
Braised Squid, 57
Creamy Clams, 58
Shrimp, Mussels and Clams Appetizer, 91
Coconut Crab Spread, 95
Mussels and Veggies Appetizer, 96
Octopus Salad, 103
Clams and Mussels Appetizer Salad, 107

SESAME
Zucchini Hummus, 98

SHALLOTS
Salmon Salad, 104
Strawberry Dip, 106

CHILI
Chili Dip

SHRIMPS
Delicious Shrimp, 48
Garlic Shrimp, 48
Shrimp and Squash Mix, 49
Shrimp Stew, 53
Italian Shrimp, 55
Shrimp, Mussels and Clams Appetizer, 91
Curried Shrimp Appetizer, 91
Stuffed Mushrooms, 99
Creole Shrimp Appetizer, 102

SPINACH
Tasty Spinach Quiche, 10
Spinach and Feta Quiche, 15
Burrito Bowls, 23
Spinach and Squash Mix, 60
Summer Greenie Mix, 62
Creamy Spinach, 67

140

Balsamic Spinach and Chard, 72
Spanish Spinach Mix, 81
Spinach and Chestnut Dip, 87
Stuffed Chicken Breast Appetizer, 92

SQUASH
Squash and Zucchini Pudding, 25
Butternut Squash Mix, 31
Beef and Veggie Stew, 40
Shrimp and Squash Mix, 49
Mexican Veggie Mix, 59
Spinach and Squash Mix, 60
Special Cauliflower Rice Mix, 61
Squash and Parsnips Mix, 62
Summer Greenie Mix, 62
Zucchini and Squash Side Dish, 65
Squash Mash, 73
Squash and Cauliflower Spread, 85
Radish Dip, 104
Squash Dessert, 114
Squash Pudding, 133

STRAWBERRIES
Sour Apples and Strawberries Breakfast Mix, 32
Strawberry Dip, 106
Mascarpone and Berries Cream, 110
Berries Marmalade, 113
Strawberries and Blueberries Marmalade, 118
Sweet Strawberry Cream, 121
Strawberry Marmalade, 130

TOMATOES
Italian Eggs, 14
Incredible Turkey and Bacon Casserole, 14
Tomatoes Casserole, 23
Burrito Bowls, 23
Fajita Bowls, 28
Breakfast Veggies Mix, 30
Delicious Pork Chili, 34
Chili Verde, 37
Tasty Meatballs, 41
Beef Tongue Mix, 44
Ground Beef Soup, 44
Delicious Shrimp, 48
Simple Oxtail Stew, 49
Shrimp Stew, 53
Tasty Seafood Stew, 54
Fall Veggie Mix, 63
Cherry Tomatoes Side Dish, 73
Broccoli and Tomatoes Mix, 76
Collard Greens, Bacon and Tomatoes, 79
Squash and Swiss Chard Mix, 82
Simple Cherry Tomatoes and Onion Mix, 82
Creamy Eggplant and Tomatoes, 83

Eggplant and Tomato Salsa, 85
Mixed Veggies Spread, 86
Mushroom and Bell Peppers Spread, 88
Veggie Party Mix, 94
Tomato and Sweet Onion Dip, 95
Mussels and Veggies Appetizer, 96
Zucchini and Tomato Dip, 97

TURKEY
Creamy Eggs and Turkey Mix, 9
Delicious Egg Scramble, 12
Incredible Turkey and Bacon Casserole, 14
Turkey Casserole, 15
Spicy Turkey and Eggs Mix, 16
Mexican Pork Breakfast, 18
Leek, Kale and Turkey Breakfast, 29
Turkey, Cranberries and Cauliflower Bowls, 33
Rabbit Stew, 50
Shrimp Stew, 53
Cheese Dip, 96

WALNUTS
Spicy Nuts Mix, 93
Walnuts and Pumpkin Seeds Snack, 94

ZUCCHINI
Salami and Eggs Casserole, 19
Delicious Chicken Frittata, 22
Squash and Zucchini Pudding, 25
Breakfast Veggies Mix, 30
Ground Beef Soup, 44
Mexican Veggie Mix, 59
Fresh Veggie Side Dish, 59
Zucchini and Squash Side Dish, 65
Veggie Party Mix, 94
Mussels and Veggies Appetizer, 96
Zucchini and Tomato Dip, 97
Zucchini Hummus, 98
Zucchini and Cheese Rolls, 100
Zucchini Cake, 113

Copyright 2017 by Marta Getty All rights reserved.

All rights Reserved. No part of this publication or the information in it may be quoted from or reproduced in any form by means such as printing, scanning, photocopying or otherwise without prior written permission of the copyright holder.

Disclaimer and Terms of Use: Effort has been made to ensure that the information in this book is accurate and complete, however, the author and the publisher do not warrant the accuracy of the information, text and graphics contained within the book due to the rapidly changing nature of science, research, known and unknown facts and internet. The Author and the publisher do not hold any responsibility for errors, omissions or contrary interpretation of the subject matter herein. This book is presented solely for motivational and informational purposes only.

Made in the USA
Lexington, KY
19 February 2019